KT-567-366

Clinician's Guide To Nuclear Medicine

Oncology

Jamshed B. Bomanji MBBS, MSc, PhD
Consultant and Senior Lecturer
Institute of Nuclear Medicine
UCL Medical School
The Middlesex Hospital
London, UK

Keith E. Britton MD, MSc, FRCR, FRCP
Professor of Nuclear Medicine
St Bartholomew's Hospital
London, UK

Susan E. M. Clarke MBBS, MSc, FRCP
Consultant and Senior Lecturer
Department of Nuclear Medicine
United Medical and Dental Schools of
Guy's and St Thomas's Hospitals,
London, UK

© British Nuclear Medicine Society
All rights reserved; no part of this publication may be
reproduced, stored in a retrieval system, or transmitted in any
form or by any means, electronic, mechanical, photocopying,
recording or otherwise, without either the prior written
permission of the British Nuclear Medicine Society or a licence
permitting restricted copying in the United Kingdom issued by
the Copyright Licensing Agency Ltd, 32-34 Alfred Place,
London WC1E 7DP.

First published/Edition 1995

ISBN 0 901259 11 X

Presented with the compliments of
Amersham International plc
as a service to medical education.

⟁mersham **HEALTHCARE**

Preface

On behalf of the British Nuclear Medicine Society (BNMS) we began editing a series of books entitled "A Clinicians Guide to Nuclear Medicine" which intends to present the clinical utility of nuclear medicine to all doctors, whether in general medicine, surgery or special disciplines. The first three books in this series were published in 1991 and addressed the topics of brain blood flow in neurology and psychiatry, gastroenterology and benign and malignant bone disease.

We are now in a position to publish and complete this series with three further books addressing the topics of cardiology, oncology and nephrourology.

The authors of this specific book on oncology have over the years shown a particular interest in the application of nuclear medicine and the radioactive tracer principle to clinical oncology.

Nuclear medicine therapy in oncology continues to expand, beyond its routine role in the management of patients with thyroid cancer. Palliation of bone pain is now a main application with advances being made in the treatment of neural crest tumours, antibody therapy of lymphomas, and even treatment of high grade gliomas. In the diagnostic assessment of a patient with cancer, nuclear medicine is also expanding its utility. Breast imaging has become an interesting new topic, receptor imaging is gaining wide acceptability and efforts are now being made to contribute to the assessment of the patient vis a vis response to radiotherapy and/or chemotherapy.

This book describes in a succinct manner, the main areas of application of nuclear medicine to oncology.

The British Nuclear Medicine Society appreciates a significant grant from Amersham International plc which is making the publication of these three new books in this series possible.

Professor P.J. Ell, Series Editor.

ACKNOWLEDGEMENT

We would like to thank our staff members for their excellent technical support and high quality work. We are grateful to our clinical colleagues from various departments for their support and interest in this field. Special thanks to Professor Peter J. Ell for his enthusiasm and guidance in bringing this monologue to fruition.

This book is part of a series sponsored by Amersham International plc for which the authors, editor and the British Nuclear Medicine Society are grateful.

Contents

Introduction

Nuclear medicine finds cancer and in some cases treats cancer. In patients with cancer, diagnostic imaging is directed towards localisation of the primary tumour and delineation of the extent of disease. After a firm histological diagnosis has been established, imaging may further assist in directing treatment, monitoring response to therapy and detecting recurrence. These complex imaging needs of cancer patients often require multimodality imaging.

Nuclear medicine techniques (scintigraphy) largely provide functional information, which complements the morphological information obtained from radiology. These two types of data can be integrated in a modern way by viewing images of the suspected cancer site from each modality in parallel or, indeed, by co-registration of images, whereby the images from one modality are superimposed on those from another. The importance of a small abnormality on a nuclear medicine image is greatly enhanced if it can be shown to co-locate to a normal gland or a node, or a particular abnormality on x-ray computed tomography (CT) or magnetic resonance imaging (MRI). For example, in a patient with treated lymphoma, a small residual hilar mass seen on CT does not always imply active disease. However, uptake of gallium-67 (^{67}Ga) in this area would do so. Thus, the progress of nuclear medicine in oncology depends on finding that which is not clinically or radiologically evident, or demonstrating as specifically as possible the nature of a radiological abnormality. Tissue characterisation is the way forward in this endeavour.

The scintigraphic approach takes advantage of tumour-specific or associated radiopharmaceuticals for the diagnosis, staging and follow-up of disease. For this purpose specific metabolic characteristics and biological properties of the tumour are exploited. The active uptake of iodine-131 (^{131}I) through the iodine trap into thyroid cancer (provided there is no competing normal thyroid tissue) provided the first example of nuclear medicine identifying cancer tissue. Since then, numerous radionuclides and radiopharmaceuticals with different tumour uptake mechanisms have been used to identify several cancers (Table 1.1).

The last two decades have produced new, more tumour-specific radiopharmaceuticals which have crossed the bridge between research and routine clinical imaging. The specificity of tissue characterisation in malignant disease is progressing from agents such as gallium-67 (^{67}Ga) which react with both inflammatory and malignant tissue, to selective radiolabelled neuropeptides, to radiolabelled monoclonal antibodies. It is the binder-bindee concept that has enabled the considerable progress of nuclear medicine in oncology to occur. The binder-bindee may be a monoclonal antibody (MoAb) such as technetium-99m (^{99m}Tc) antimelanoma antibody, which binds to a specific antigen expressed by melanoma cells. It may be a radiolabelled peptide analogue such as octreotide (indium-111 pentetreotide), which reacts with several cancers that express the somatostatin receptor. It may also be a molecule which structurally resembles a neuro-transmitter, e.g. iodine-123 metaiodobenzylguanidine (^{123}I-MIBG) which resembles noradrenaline (Table 1.2).

Nuclear medicine is at its best when it is asked to address clinical problems which cannot be accurately resolved by other imaging modalities, e.g. demonstrating tumour recurrences before serum markers are elevated and locating them when serum markers are elevated using radiolabelled MoAbs or their fragments. Predicting response to chemotherapy is another indication which is gaining popularity. For example, it has been shown that a measure of the uptake of radiolabelled 5–fluorouracil (^{18}F-5-FU) in patients with colorectal liver metastases can predict the response to conventional 5-FU chemotherapy. High uptake of radiolabelled ^{18}F-5-FU in the metastases predicts a good response. Finally, nuclear medicine techniques are also used to monitor organ function and detect injury secondary to cancer therapy.

Diffusion	^{99m}Tc-DTPA
Diffusion and binding	^{99m}Tc-MIBI
Lipophilicity	^{99m}Tc-HMPAO
Active transport	^{131}I ^{201}Tl ^{18}F-FDG ^{123}I-methyl tyrosine
Receptor binding	^{111}In-pentetreotide ^{99m}Tc-Interleukin ^{123}I vasoactive intestinal peptide
Receptor and storage	^{123}I-MIBG
Antigen	Radiolabelled monoclonal antibodies Molecular recognition units

Table 1.1 *Mechanism of tumour uptake*

Non-specific	More specific	Class specific	Type specific
Tumour or inflammation	Tumour not inflammation	Several tumours	Few tumours
Gallium-67	Thallium-201 MoAb	Radiolabelled MoAb - anti-CEA	Radiolabelled - anti-lymphoma
^{18}F-FDG	^{99m}Tc-MIBI B72.3 MoAb	- anti-squamous - anti-neuroblastoma - PR1A3 for colorectal cancer	- anti-melanoma
'octreotide'	^{123}I-MIBG	^{123}I-IBZM	
	^{123}I/^{111}In	^{123}I-VIP	

Table 1.2 *Tissue characterisation in malignant disease*

3

Radionuclide measurements of ventricular wall motion, ejection fraction, and glomerular filtration rate are commonly used to determine cardiotoxic and nephrotoxic effects of cancer therapy.

RADIONUCLIDE THERAPY

Virtually all the imaging procedures outlined above can be converted with greater or lesser success to radionuclide therapy. The more selective and specific the uptake, the better targeted the therapy. These features are particularly responsible for the success of ^{131}I therapy of thyroid cancers and their metastases and ^{131}I-MIBG therapy of neural crest tumours, in particular neuroblastoma. Therapeutic effect depends on the release of beta particles (electrons) from the radionuclide which liberate a considerable amount of destructive energy over a short path length of not more than a centimetre in tissue. This targeting has advantages over external beam radiotherapy in that it is the specific tumour cells that are targeted. However, it has a major disadvantage inasmuch as a significant amount of the radionuclide-labelled compound is distributed in normal tissues. Therefore, in order to obtain a good therapeutic ratio it is necessary for the unbound radiolabelled material to be cleared rapidly from the body. The lessons that can be learnt from ^{131}I therapy of thyroid cancer for newer forms of radionuclide therapy are set out in Table 1.3. The longer the residence time of the radionuclide therapy on the tumour and the shorter the residence time in the normal tissues of the body, the greater the therapeutic ratio. Thus longer-lived beta imaging radionuclides such as phosphorus-32 (^{32}P) (14.3-day half-life) strontium-89 (^{89}Sr) (50.5-day half-life) and indium-114m ([114m]In) (60-day half-life) are being evaluated. However, if the therapeutic radiation has to be delivered to the tissue before the radionuclide therapy compound escapes into the bloodstream from its particular site, such as a joint or the peritoneum, then a short-lived radionuclide in high dose is required such as yttrium-90 (^{90}Y) (2.7-day half-life), samarium-153 ([153]Sm) (3-day half-life) or rhenium ([186]Re)

• Confirmation of *in vivo* tumour uptake before therapy
• Avoidance of interfering drugs
• Use of a long-lived beta-emitting radionuclide: ^{131}I   8 days ^{32}P   14.3 days ^{89}Sr   50.5 days
• Use of high activity not repeated earlier than 6 months
• The rapid excretion pathway to reduce normal tissue irradiation
• Avoidance of immunosuppression to allow a normal immunological response to radio-damaged cells

Table 1.3 *Lessons from ^{131}I therapy*

(3.8–day half-life). A selection of radionuclide therapies is given in Table 1.4.

In conclusion, nuclear medicine techniques contribute significant functional information. They add specificity and tissue characterisation to their sensitivity in detecting malignant disease and aim to provide better management of patients with cancer.

[131]I	Thyroid cancer
[89]Sr	Bone metastases from prostate and breast cancer
[153]Sm EDTMP	Bone metastases
[186]Re HEDP	Bone metastases
[131]I MIBG	Neuroblastoma
	Malignant paragangliomas
	Carcinoid
[131]I-labelled MoAb	Malignant effusions and ascites (intracavitary) Intratumour and intravenous therapy for cancer
[131]I-Lipiodol	Hepatoma (Intra-arterial)
[90]Y-labelled MoAb	Intraperitoneal therapy for ovarian cancer Two stage therapy for cancer
[32]P phosphate	Polycythaemia rubra vera Thrombocythaemia
[32]P chromic phosphate	Intracerebral tumour therapy
[32]P colloids	Malignant effusions
[186]Re-DMSA(V)	Medullary thyroid carcinoma
[114m]In A31 cells	Lymphoma

Key:
MoAb, tumour-associated monoclonal antibodies.
EDTMP and HEDP, bone-seeking phosphate derivatives.
DMSA (V), dimercaptosuccinic acid (alkaline).
MIBG, metaiodobenzylguanidine.

Table 1.4 *Radionuclide therapy for cancer*

Lymphomas

INTRODUCTION

Lymphomas are the result of malignant transformations of T cells or B cells. They are usually divided into Hodgkin's or non-Hodgkin's lymphoma. In both, it is important to establish the extent of the disease as the choice of therapy depends on accurate knowledge of the stage of the disease. In this context, laboratory and imaging investigations are used and diagnostic studies undertaken to monitor response to therapy and detect recurrence.

The Cotswald Staging Classification for Hodgkin's Disease[1]

Stage I. Involvement of a single lymph node region.

Stage II. Involvement of two or more lymph node regions on the same side of the diaphragm.

Stage III. Involvement of lymph node regions on both sides of the diaphragm.

Stage IV. Multifocal involvement of one or more extralymphatic organs with or without lymph node involvement.

Conventional diagnostic radiology, computed tomography (CT) and ultrasonography (US) give information about tumour size and distribution of lesions. However, these imaging techniques do not adequately reflect changes such as fibrosis and tumour necrosis. A residual mediastinal mass, for instance, does not necessarily indicate active disease, and this represents a common and difficult diagnostic problem.

After the history and examination, chest x-ray and routine blood counts are completed and after the diagnosis is confirmed by lymph node biopsy, staging is normally undertaken by a

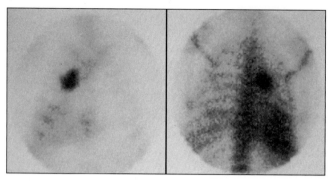

Fig. 2.1 *Hodgkin's disease imaged with* ^{67}*Ga. Planar images: left panel shows anterior chest and right panel posterior chest. There is a large focal area of increased uptake in the right upper chest compatible with an active recurrence of Hodgkin's disease in the mediastinum*

whole-body x-ray CT scan. Lymph nodes larger than 1 or 1.5 cm depending on different investigators' criteria, are designated as involved nodes and the staging is made on this basis.

NUCLEAR MEDICINE INVESTIGATIONS

The purpose of nuclear medicine investigations is to facilitate staging and to aid in determining viability of residual nodal disease after chemotherapy or radiotherapy. In particular lymph nodes demonstrated by x-ray CT that are less than 1cm in diameter may be shown by nuclear medicine techniques to contain viable tumour.

A large variety of scintigraphic techniques are now available for imaging these tumours. Traditionally ^{67}Ga along with ^{99m}Tc–MDP bone scintigraphy was considered as part of the staging protocol for these tumours. The role of bone scanning has been discussed previously[2] and will not be addressed in this series.

Gallium-67

Gallium-67 is a gamma-emitting radionuclide with three main gamma energies and a half-life of 78 h. ^{67}Ga binds to transferrin protein in the blood and transferrin receptors on cells including white cells and tumours. Because of its natural secretion into the lumen of the bowel it is not recommended for studies below the diaphragm. Bowel preparation and laxatives make little difference.

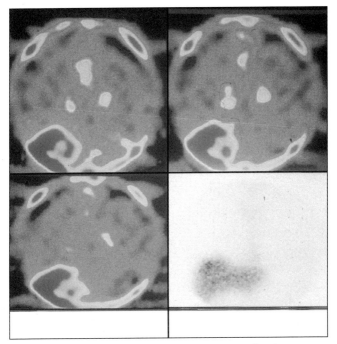

Fig. 2.2 *Hodgkin's disease imaged with* ^{67}*Ga. Bottom right: planar image of the anterior chest which is normal. Top left, top right, bottom left: serial coronal sections demonstrating uptake in two mediastinal nodes each side of the midline. There is also uptake in the manubrium sterni seen in the top left image, and in the liver. SPET can reveal sites of abnormal uptake not evident on planar imaging with high-dose* ^{67}*Ga*

It should be remembered that ^{67}Ga is a non-specific agent. It is taken up in a variety of tumours and infections. Therefore it is best that ^{67}Ga studies are either undertaken properly, seriously and serially or not at all. A baseline ^{67}Ga study is performed prior to any treatment and a follow-up scan is performed after termination of treatment.

It is recommended that scintigraphy should be performed with a high dose (370 MBq) of ^{67}Ga and planar images should be performed at 48 h and 72 h post-injection (Fig. 2.1). For assessment of residual mediastinal disease, SPET imaging should be performed as it increases the sensitivity for detection (Fig. 2.2). Essentially no patient preparation is required for this investigation.

9

The images must be compared with the CT scan of the thorax and abnormalities must be identified on all three orthogonal planes on SPET and related to the x-ray CT findings. Studies performed with high-dose ^{67}Ga SPET imaging have reported sensitivity ranging between 85% and 92%[3,4]. In a recent study of 99 treated lymphoma patients it was shown that scintigraphy was a better predictor of disease-free survival than CT[5]. False–negative scans may be obtained if ^{67}Ga scintigraphy is performed too soon after therapy. In our experience, ^{67}Ga uptake 7-9 weeks after therapy is a reliable indicator for active disease.

[111]In-[DTPA-D-Phe[1]]-octreotide (^{111}In-pentetreotide)

Recently it was shown that lymphomas (Hodgkin's and non-Hodgkin's) express somatostatin receptors[6,7,8]. The presence of these receptors on the tumours provides the possibility of imaging them with radiolabelled somatostatin analogues such as ^{111}In-pentetreotide. This radiopharmaceutical is taken up by a variety of tumours and lymphomas but not usually by infections (see Chap. on Gastroendocrine Tumours for further details). A recent study has shown that ^{111}In-pentetreotide is better suited to characterise somatostatin receptor-expressing lymphomas than to localise lesion sites[9]. The reported sensitivity of detecting Hodgkin's disease was 70% and varied from 88% in the neck and chest to 13% in the abdomen and pelvis. For non-Hodgkin's lymphoma the sensitivity was 35%.

Radiolabelled monoclonal antibodies

Both B- and T-cell lymphocytes have a wide range of important molecular markers on their surface. These are known by their CD numbers. Monoclonal antibodies against CD3 and CD4 react with T-cell and T-cell-derived tumours. Those against CD19 to CD37 react with a variety of B-cell tumours. It has been difficult to produce a monoclonal antibody which reacts with Hodgkin's disease, although the new agent LL2[10] shows promise. Monoclonal antibodies have been labelled progressively

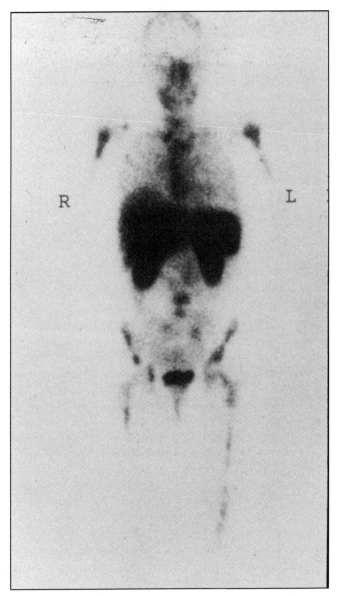

Fig. 2.3 *Non-Hodgkin's lymphoma. Anterior view of the whole body. Multiple lymph node and marrow involvement imaged using ^{99m}Tc-LL2, a monoclonal antibody. (Courtesy of Dr David Goldenberg)*

with ^{131}I, ^{111}In, ^{123}I and ^{99m}Tc (Fig. 2.3). These agents have been
used for diagnosis of non-Hodgkin's lymphoma. ^{131}I-monoclonal
antibodies such as LYM-1 and LL-2, have been used for the
therapy of non-Hodgkin's lymphoma. ^{131}I-anti-CD37 (MB-1) and
^{131}I-anti-CD20(B1) have been the most successful[11,12]. Whereas
high- or medium-grade non-Hodgkin's lymphoma tends to
respond well to chemotherapy, the low-grade non-Hodgkin's
lymphoma, although responding to therapy initially, tends to be
slowly progressive. It is to this end that both diagnosis and
therapy with radiolabelled monoclonal antibodies are targeted.
Hodgkin's lymphoma has been treated with ^{131}I-antiferritin in
combination with chemotherapy[13]. Success in the imaging and
therapy of hairy cell leukaemia, which often presents with lymph
node involvement, has been achieved using an antibody T-101
labelled with ^{131}I.

^{18}F-Fluorodeoxyglucose (^{18}F-FDG) PET imaging

^{18}F-FDG is a sugar analogue, 2-deoxyglucose, labelled with a
positron emitter Fluorine-18. The accumulation of ^{18}F-FDG is
based on the intracellular trapping of ^{18}F-FDG 6-phosphate,
which is the product of the hexokinase reaction on FDG.
Further metabolism of FDG 6-phosphate is restricted in tissue
devoid of glucose 6-phosphatase due to steric inhibition of
enzyme activities by the fluorine atom in position 2 of the
glucal ring. Thus increased radioactivity will be detected in
tissues that have a high glucose utilisation and lack of glucose
6-phosphatase, such as malignant tissues. In small pilot studies
using this radiopharmaceutical, malignant lymphomas have
been successfully imaged (Fig. 2.4)[14,15].

This glucose analogue is taken up by active tissue: tumour
cells, macrophages, bacterial infections and granuloma.
In tumours, the malignant process increases the production of
the glucose 1 transporter protein, so ^{18}F-FDG enters in
increased amount into tumour cells. Then it is phosphorylated
by the hexokinase enzyme, whereby further metabolism is
blocked. It does not enter the pathway of aerobic or anaerobic
metabolism. Since viable cells in their growth phase take up
glucose it may be used, like ^{67}Ga, as an indicator of viable
lymphoma when CT scans show enlarged or suspicious

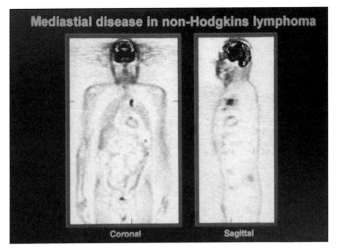

Fig. 2.4 *Non-Hodgkin's lymphoma imaged with ^{18}F-FDG PET. Coronal and sagittal views of the whole body show a focal area of increased tracer uptake in the mediastinal region compatible with residual disease*

lymph nodes. The cyclotron production and the specialised imaging equipment are very expensive, but whole body PET is competitive with serial slice CT imaging in this context. Its contribution to the management of such patients should soon be established.

^{201}Tl, ^{99m}Tc-MIBI

^{201}Tl and ^{99m}Tc-MIBI have also been used for imaging lymphomas [16,17]. It has been shown that for low grade lymphomas both radiopharmaceuticals are superior to ^{67}Ga. However, large prospective studies are required to further support this data.

References

1. Lister TA, Crowther D, Sutcliffe SB et al. Report of a committee convened to discuss the evaluation and staging of patients with Hodgkin's disease: Cotswald meeting. *J of Clin Oncology* 1989; **7**: 1630-1636; *J of Clin Oncology* [Erratum] 1990; **8**: 1602.

2. McKillop JH, Fogelman I. Oncology. In, Benign and malignant bone disease. *Churchill Livingstone*, London 1991; 30-52.

3. Tumeh SS, Rosenthal DS, Kaplan WD, English RJ, Holman LB. Lymphoma: evaluation wih Ga-67 SPECT. *Radiology* 1987; **164**: 111-114.

4. Front D, Israel O, Epelbaum R, et al. Ga-67 SPECT before and after treatment of lymphoma. *Radiology* 1990; **175**: 515-519.

5. Front D, Ben-Haim S, Israel O, et al. Lymphoma: Predictive value of Ga-67 scintigraphy after treatment. *Radiology* 1992; **182**: 359-363.

6. Lamberts SWJ, Krenning EP, Reubi JC. The role of somatostatin and its analogs in the diagnosis and treatment of tumours. *Endocrine Reviews* 1991; **12**: 450-482.

7. Vaanhagen PM, Krenning EP, Reubi JC, et al. Somatostatin analogue scintigraphy of malignant lymphomas. *Brit. J. Haematology* 1992; **82**: 75-79.

8. Krenning EP, Kwekkeboom DJ, Bakker WH, et al. Somatostatin receptor scintigraphy with ^{111}In-DTPA-d-Phe[1] and ^{123}I-Tyr[3]-octreotide: Rotterdam experience with more than 1000 patients. *European J. of Nuclear Medicine* 1993; **20**: 716-731.

9. Lipp RW, Silly H, Ranner G, et al. Radiolabelled octreotide for the demonstration of somatostatin receptors in malignant lymphoma and lymphadenopathy. *J. of Nuclear Medicine* 1995; **36**: 13-18.

10. Goldenberg DM, Sharkey RM, Juweid AL, et al. Imaging, targeting and therapy of non-Hodgkin's lymphoma with radiolabelled LL2 murine and chimeric monoclonal antibodies. *European J. of Nuclear Medicine* 1994; **21**: S24.

11. Kaminsky MS, Zasadny KR, Francis IR, et al. Radioimmunotherapy of B-cell lymphoma with [^{131}I] anti-B1 (antiCD20) antibody. *New England J. of Medicine* 1993; **329**: 459-465.

12. Press OW, Eary JF, Appelbaum FR, et al. Radiolabelled-antibody therapy of B-cell lymphoma with autologous bone marrow support. *New England J. of Medicine* 1993; **329**: 1219-1224.

13. Order SE, Klein JL, Ettinger D, et al. ^{131}I-antiferritin: a new treatment modality in hepatoma: a Radiation Therapy Oncology Group. *J. of Clinical Oncology* 1985; **3**: 1573–1582.

14. Paul R. Comparison of fluorine-18-2-fluorodeoxyglucose and gallium-67 citrate imaging for detection of lymphoma. *J. of Nuclear Medicine* 1987; **28**: 288-292.

15. Okada J, Yoshikawa K, Imazeki K, et al. The use of FDG-PET in the detection and management of malignant lymphoma: correlation of uptake and prognosis. *J. of Nuclear Medicine* (1991); **32**: 686-691.

16. Waxman AD, Ramanna L, Eller D. Characterization of lymphoma grade using thallium and gallium scintigraphy. *J. of Nuclear Medicine* (1991), **32**: 917-918

17. Waxman AD, Nagaraj N, Khan S, Heifetz L, McAndrews P, Bierman H, Avedon M. Tc-99m sestamibi (MIBI) in the evaluation of lymphoma: comparison with gallium-67 citrate. *J. of Nuclear Medicine* (1995), **36**: 117.

Thyroid Cancer

INTRODUCTION

Radionuclides play an important part in all aspects of thyroid cancer management. Currently thyroid imaging is performed for the evaluation of a palpable nodule using an intravenous injection of [123]I (20 MBq) or [99m]TcO₄ (80 MBq). [131]I in diagnostic doses is commonly used for imaging patients with thyroid cancers, while large doses are used for therapeutic purposes. [131]I is also used when a retrosternal goitre needs to be differentiated from a more sinister mass which might require exploratory surgery. To obtain good-quality images and quantitative data the patient must be free of iodine and other competing compounds such as iodine contrast media and iodine in medicines, since they interfere with the uptake mechanism of the tracer (Table 3.1).

Evaluation of a clinically solitary Thyroid Nodule

The initial steps in a patient with a thyroid nodule are to obtain a careful history and to perform a physical examination to identify recognised risk factors and signs indicating malignancy. Initial imaging of the nodule requires a thyroid scan. If the palpable nodule proves to be a functional nodule ('hot' nodule) then the chances of an underlying malignancy are remote[1]. If the nodule is 'cold' then it should be further evaluated by ultrasonography, which helps to differentiate between cystic and solid lesions[2]. This should be combined with aspiration cytology for nodules less than 4 cm and cutting-needle biopsy for the echogenic nodule larger than 4 cm. Several groups have shown a reduction in surgery rate for nodules (ranging from 25-60%) as a consequence of routine fine-needle aspiration biopsy of cold nodules[3,4]. Fine-needle aspiration biopsy has become the initial test in most patients. On its own it can give false-negative results,

• Antithyroid medications:	carbimazole and propylthiouracil
• Iodide-containing medications:	Lugol's iodine, potassium iodide (and iodate), numerous vitamin preparations, antiparasitic drugs
• Thyroid replacement:	thyroxine, liothyronine, thyroid extracts
• Radiographic contrast media:	
• Other medication:	amiodarone, perchlorate, adrenocorticosteroids, anticoagulants, cimetidine, salicylates (large doses) sulfonamides, and heavy metals.
• Skin preparations:	Tincture iodine used for surgery
• Henna hair dye and skin lotions containing iodine	

Table 3.1 *Medications which interfere with iodine uptake*

but in combination with ultrasound and thyroid scintigraphy it is safe and leads to a better selection of patients for surgery than any other test[5].

The majority of thyroid cancers (80%) are well-differentiated follicular (~ 15%) or papillary carcinomas (~ 65%). Approximately 5% are medullary tumours and 5-15% are anaplastic and other tumours[6]. Cancer tends to be found more often in patients who have a solitary nodule on physical examination, although many patients may actually have multiple nodules when imaging or surgical procedures are done[7]. Approximately 6-20% of solitary cold nodules are malignant[8]. The remaining 'cold' nodules consist of degenerative nodules, haemorrhage, cysts (Fig. 3.1), inflammatory nodules (e.g. Hashimoto's thyroiditis), non–thyroidal tumours and infiltrative disorders (e.g. amyloid). The incidence of cancer in one of the nodules of multinodular goitre is lower than in a solitary nodule, but the risk of cancer in such a lesion is still sufficiently high that

17

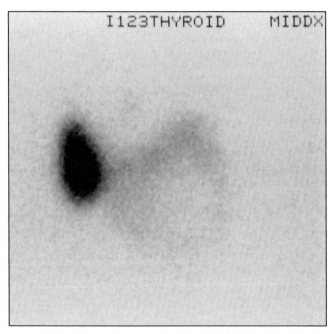

Fig. 3.1 *Thyroid image in a patient with a palpable thyroid nodule in the left thyroid lobe. The scan shows an area of deficient tracer uptake ('cold' nodule) corresponding to the palpable nodule. The rest of the gland shows normal homogeneous tracer uptake. Ultrasonography confirmed that the nodule was cystic in nature*

needle biopsy is warranted for hypo-functioning lesions that are dominant, hard or rapidly growing. Patients who have had previous external radiation to the head and neck regions have a higher incidence of benign and malignant thyroid nodules and have a 40% chance of having a thyroid cancer. The probability of malignancy is also increased in patients with Graves' disease but with a cold nodule on scintigraphy[7]. All such nodules should be considered for excision[5].

Medullary thyroid cancer (MTC) arises from the C cells of the gland, which are of neural crest origin. Unlike papillary and follicular cancer, MTC does not metabolize iodine, nor does it produce thyroglobulin, but it does secrete calcitonin. Medullary

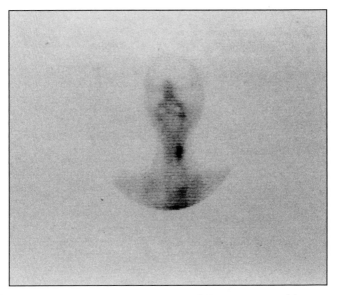

Fig. 3.2 *Lymph node metastases from medullary carcinoma of the thyroid imaged with ^{99m}Tc-dimercaptosuccinic acid (DMSA-V). The images were taken 4 h after intravenous injection of ^{99m}Tc-DMSA (V). Note the focal uptake in the left cervical chain of lymph nodes. (Courtesy of Dr. I. Datseris)*

carcinoma of the thyroid, which on a conventional thyroid scan appears as a defect (cold area), may be imaged using ^{99m}Tc–pentavalent dimercaptosuccinic acid [DMSA (V)] (Fig. 3.2), ^{201}Tl, ^{123}I-MIBG and ^{111}In-pentetreotide, which show increased tracer uptake at the tumour site[7,9,10]. The sensitivity of tumour detection with ^{99m}Tc-DMSA (V) is 78%, with ^{201}Tl, 71%, with ^{123}I-MIBG, 35% and with ^{111}In-pentetreotide, 66%.

Medullary carcinomas associated with multiple endocrine neoplasia (MEN) types 2A and 2B are frequently bilateral and multifocal. In this setting the index of suspicion for thyroid malignancy must be high, but measurement of stimulated calcitonin levels is the procedure of choice and serial gamma camera imaging has little utility.

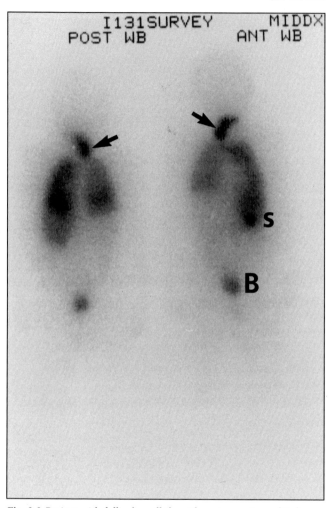

Fig. 3.3 *Patient with follicular cell thyroid carcinoma imaged 3 days after diagnostic dose of* ^{131}*I. The image shows irregular and increased tracer uptake in the paratracheal region (arrow) and diffuse high lung uptake. Such uptake may occur rarely when there is a normal chest x-ray, but usually this is associated with miliary lung metastases. B = normal excretion of tracer in bladder. S = normal gastric activity*

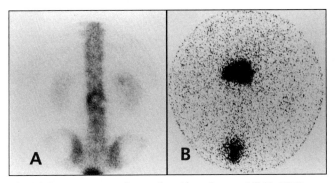

Fig. 3.4 *Bone metastases from a thyroid carcinoma. A ^{99m}Tc-MDP bone scan shows a photon-deficient area in lumbar spine. B ^{131}I diagnostic scan shows increased tracer uptake in the spine corresponding to the photon-deficient area seen on the bone scan, confirming that the bone metastases show avidity for ^{131}I*

Role of ^{131}I in Metastatic Thyroid Cancer

Approximately 80% of metastases from well-differentiated thyroid cancer take up ^{131}I provided normal thyroid tissue has been ablated. Medullary thyroid cancers, anaplastic tumours and lymphomas of the thyroid do not show any avidity for ^{131}I. Recurrence of the well-differentiated cancers occurs in approximately 21% of patients. Recurrences are more frequent at the extremes of age (<20 and >59 years) and with tumours larger than 1.5 cm that are locally invasive or metastatic. They involve the neck alone in 79%, while distant metastases account for the rest. Cervical and mediastinal lymph node metastases occur more frequently with papillary than with follicular thyroid carcinoma (46% versus 25%)[11].

Distant metastases from well-differentiated thyroid cancers commonly involve a) lung alone 63%, b) bone alone 19% and c) multiple sites 19%[11]. Metastatic spread to bones and lungs occurs more frequently in patients with follicular carcinoma of the thyroid (FCT) than in those with papillary cancers. Unfortunately, lung metastases concentrate radioiodine only in approximately 50% of patients with FCT (Fig. 3.3). On the other hand, although bone metastases usually do concentrate radioiodine (Fig 3.4), they frequently do not respond in a

21

clinically meaningful manner, despite repeated seemingly adequate therapeutic doses. Hence, other adjuvant modalities are sometimes used in the management of metastatic, persistent or recurrent disease.

Well-differentiated FCT rarely causes hyperthyroidism. The clinical presentation is similar to Graves' disease except that evidence of metastatic disease is often present (soft tissue masses and bone pain). The metastases are in the usual location and are often bulky. Despite the poor efficiency of iodine uptake and thyroid hormone production, the large tumour mass is capable of producing excessive hormone.

Ovarian teratoma (struma ovarii) is another condition associated with thyrotoxicosis in about 25% of cases. Approximately 5-10% of struma ovarii contain malignant thyroid tissue which has an avidity for ^{131}I and are treated with surgical resection followed by ^{131}I radiotherapy.

Hurthle cell (or oxyphil cell) carcinoma is an uncommon form of thyroid cancer that is usually classified as a variant of FCT. Generally there is lack of ^{131}I uptake by the metastases. Nevertheless, occasionally positive uptake can be demonstrated and subsequent treatment with ^{131}I has proved beneficial.

Post-ablation ^{131}I Follow-up Scans

^{131}I scanning is an important follow-up investigation in patients with well-differentiated thyroid cancers. It must be judiciously applied to carefully prepared and selected patients. The amount of ^{131}I employed for diagnostic purposes should range between 185 and 550 MBq given orally. If the patient is on thyroxine (T_4) then this should be stopped 6 weeks prior to administration of ^{131}I and liothyronine (T_3) substituted. Then T_3 should be withdrawn for at least 7 days prior to the diagnostic dose of ^{131}I. During this period the patient should be on a low-iodine diet. To achieve maximum uptake in metastatic lesions, it is generally recommended that the TSH levels should be above 30 mIU/l. If further enhancement of TSH levels is required then this can be induced by giving 200 μg of TRH i.v. 20 min prior to the diagnostic dose of ^{131}I. Scanning is generally performed 72 h and 96 h post

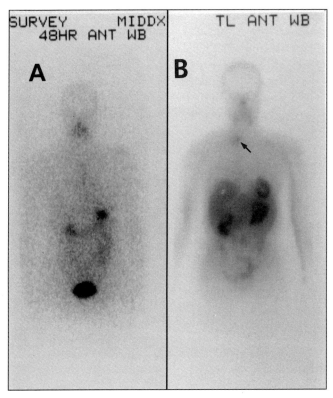

Figure 3.5 *De-differentiated follicular carcinoma of the thyroid with raised thyroglobulin levels. A Negative ^{131}I whole-body scan. B ^{201}Tl scan showing uptake in the thyroid bed corresponding to the site of recurrence (arrow)*

administration of [131]I.

It is also customary to scan the patient approximately 1 week after administration of an ablative dose of [131]I. This allows one to assess the extent of disease and in some instances may explain the failure to respond fully to the therapy dose given. The timing of the first scans after surgery and remnant ablation, as well as the intervals between scans, is arbitary and should be based upon the patient's risk for recurrent disease and distant metastases or the growth rate of known metastases.

Serum thyroglobulin measurements are useful tumour markers in patients who have had total thyroidectomy or remnant ablation with [131]I. They are an important complement to ^{131}I scanning since they predict the presence of non-functioning metastases. Metastases from differentiated papillary and follicular thyroid carcinomas are associated with a raised serum thyroglobulin level of more than 10 µg/ml in patients with an ablated gland maintained on T_4 replacement. Serum thyroglobulin levels are less useful in patients who have had limited surgery. A good review of ^{131}I and thyroid cancer is given by O'Doherty et al.[12].

Other Imaging Techniques

Both follicular and papillary carcinomas may de-differentiate over time and lose their ability to trap iodine, whilst retaining the ability to secrete thyroglobulin. Occasionally a patient may have abnormal levels of serum thyroglobulin and a negative ^{131}I scan. To circumvent this problem a ^{201}Tl or ^{99m}Tc-MIBI scan should be performed to identify metastatic sites (Fig. 3.5). Ramanna et al.[13] showed focal accumulation of ^{201}Tl along with elevated serum thyroglobulin values but normal findings on diagnostic ^{131}I scans in 29% of patients.

Rarely, a patient will present with evidence of distant metastatic disease, e.g. pathological fracture, with subsequent discovery of the thyroid tumour. Although bone is a common site for metastatic disease, screening bone scans are generally not indicated. Bone scans are useful in identifying sites of metastases in patients with known metastatic non-functioning tumour and in patients with bone pain.

References

1. Freitas JE, Gross MD, Ripley S, Shapiro B. Radionuclide diagnosis and therapy of thyroid cancer: current status report. *Seminars in Nuclear Medicine* (1985); **15**: 106-131.

2. Leisner B. Ultrasound evaluation of thyroid disease. *Hormone Research* 1987; **26**: 33-41.

3. Dumitriu L, Moqos I, Calin E. Fine needle aspiration biopsy

of the thyroid correlated with clinical scintigraphic, echographic and pathologic data in nodular and diffuse goitre. *Endocrinologie* 1984; **22**: 261-268.

4. Al Sayer HM, Krukowsi ZH, Williams VMM, Matheson NA. Fine needle aspiration cytology in isolated thyroid swellings: a prospective two year evaluation. *Brit. Med. Journal* 1985; **290**: 1490-1492.

5. Mazzaferri EL. Management of a solitary thyroid nodule. *New England J. of Medicine* 1993; **328**: 553-559.

6. Hedinger C, Williams ED, Sobin LH. The WHO histological classification of thyroid tumours: a commentary on the second edition. *Cancer* 1989: **63**: 908-911.

7. Fogelman I, Maisey MN. The thyroid scan in the management of thyroid disease. In: *Nuclear Medicine Annual,* Raven Press, New York 1989: 1-48.

8. Wesk EE, Vernon BM, Gonzalez JJ, et al. Cancer in thyroid nodules. *Archives of Int. Medicine* 1984; **144**: 474-476.

9. Clark SEM. Tumour imaging. In clinical nuclear medicine. (ed. MN Maisey, KE Britton, DL Gilday), *Chapman and Hall Medical* 1991: 426-459

10. Krenning EP, Kwekkeboom DJ, Bakker WH, et al. Somatostatin receptor scintigraphy with ^{111}In-DTPA-D-Phe1 and ^{123}I-Tyr[3]-octreotide: Rotterdam experience with more than 1000 patients. *European J. of Nuclear Medicine* 1993; **20**: 716-731.

11. Mazzaferri EL, Jhiang, SM. Long-term impact of initial surgical and medical therapy on papillary and follicular thyroid cancer. *The American J. of Medicine* 1994; **97**: 418-428.

12. O'Doherty MJ, Nunan TO, Croft DN. Radionuclides and therapy of thyroid cancer. *Nuclear Medicine Comms* 1993; **14**: 736-755.

13. Ramanna L, Waxman A, Braunstein G. Thallium-201 scintigraphy in differentiated thyroid cancer. Comparison with radioiodine scintigraphy and serum thyroglobulin determinations. *J. of Nuclear Medicine* 1991; **32**: 441-446.

Adrenal Tumours

INTRODUCTION

Imaging is an essential adjunct to the clinical and biochemical findings in the diagnosis of adrenal disorders. A carefully planned approach that considers all the available imaging techniques can, in virtually every instance, identify and efficiently localise sources of abnormal adrenal hormone production.

In the field of nuclear medicine, progress has been significant, and new radiopharmaceuticals for imaging neuroendocrine tumours have become available. The most important of these, radioiodine-labelled MIBG, is used for imaging and therapy of neural crest tumours[1,2]. ^{111}In–pentetreotide, an octreotide analogue, is another radiopharmaceutical recently developed and used for imaging tumours with somatostatin receptors[3].

[123]I-metaiodobenzylguanidine (^{123}I-MIBG) Imaging

MIBG is an aralkylguanidine which structurally resembles noradrenaline. ^{123}I-MIBG is used for imaging phaeochromocytomas (Fig. 4.1), paragangliomas (Fig. 4.2), neuroblastomas and carcinoid tumours (Fig. 4.3)[1,4,5,6]. The main indications for ^{123}I-MIBG scintigraphy are to define functionally the nature of an adrenal mass, to detect extra–adrenal lesions, to enable early detection of recurrent disease, and as an essential prelude to ^{131}I-MIBG therapy. For diagnostic imaging and therapy with radiolabelled MIBG, patient preparation is very important. Drugs which interfere with the uptake mechanism of this tracer need to be stopped[7]. Some common drugs which interfere with the uptake of this

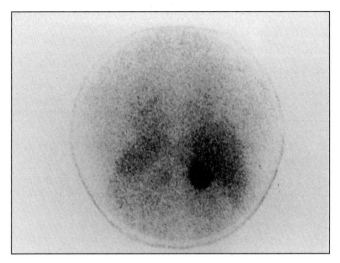

Fig. 4.1 [123]*I-MIBG posterior chest image of a patient with a phaeochromocytoma. There is focal and increased tracer uptake in the right adrenal gland (phaeochromocytoma). Outline of the normal left adrenal gland is also visualised*

tracer are outlined in Table 4.1. Prior to the scan the thyroid gland also needs to be blocked with Lugol's iodine or potassium iodide. Approximately 185-370 MBq of ^{123}I-MIBG or 20 MBq of ^{131}I-MIBG is injected intravenously and whole–body images are acquired at various time intervals.

PHAEOCHROMOCYTOMAS AND PARAGANGLIOMAS

Phaeochromocytomas and paragangliomas are catecholamine-secreting tumours of neural crest origin and are a challenge to both the surgeon and the anaesthetist. Early detection of these tumours is important because it offers the possibility of curing hypertension after surgical resection. Diagnosis generally rests on laboratory test results. Once biochemical diagnosis is confirmed, localisation of the tumour becomes mandatory. It is in this context that ^{123}I-MIBG scintigraphy is extremely useful since it has a high sensitivity (Table 4.2)[8]. In patients

27

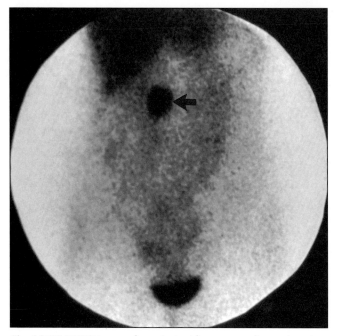

Fig. 4.2 ^{123}I-MIBG image of a patient with a paraganglioma. Anterior view of the abdomen showing a focal area of increased tracer uptake in the region of the right sympathetic chain corresponding to the site of the paraganglioma (arrow) confirmed at surgery. Normal excretion of the tracer is seen in the urinary bladder

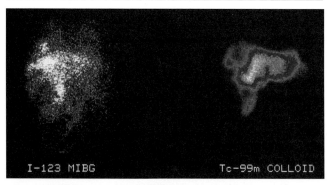

Fig. 4.3 ^{123}I-MIBG image of a patient with a metastatic carcinoid tumour. **Left panel:** ^{123}I-MIBG scan, anterior view, showing multiple areas of increased tracer uptake some of which correspond to the photon-deficient areas seen on the ^{99m}Tc colloid scan (**right panel**)

- Reserpine

- Tricyclic antidepressants

- Cocaine

- Sympathomimetics (e.g. phenylpropanolamine)

- Guanethidine

- Antipsychotics (e.g., phenothiazines)

- Calcium-channel blockers

- Over the counter medication, e.g. nose drops, ear drops and nose and throat sprays which may contain sympathomimetics

Table 4.1 *Common drugs which interfere with MIBG uptake*

Tumour type	^{123}I-MIBG	^{111}In-pentetreotide
Phaeochromocytoma	88%	88%
Paragangliomas	89%	97%
Neuroblastomas	92%	77%
Carcinoid	71%	86%
Medullary thyroid cancer	35%	66%

Hoefnagel, C.A. MIBG and somatostatin in oncology: role in the management of neural crest tumours. *European J. of Nuclear Medicine* 1994; **21**: 561-581.

Table 4.2 *Sensitivity of ^{131}I-MIBG and ^{111}In-pentetreotide in detecting neural crest tumours*

with equivocal clinical and biochemical findings for any of the aforementioned tumours, a negative ^{123}I-MIBG scan excludes the need for further investigation. If there is strong biochemical and clinical evidence for these tumours, and the ^{123}I-MIBG scan is negative, then CT of the chest, abdomen and pelvis should be performed. If ^{123}I-MIBG scan is positive, showing the primary lesion with no metastases, then tailored CT of that area should be performed to delineate accurately the mass pre–operatively. In cases where ^{123}I-MIBG shows evidence of metastatic disease, CT is unlikely to alter the clinical management unless imaging guidance is required for biopsy[4]. Generally, the degree of uptake is related to the number of chromaffin granules in the tumour. The overall sensitivity for detection of phaeochromocytomas with ^{131}I-MIBG is 88% which is similar to the sensitivity of CT and MRI. The sensitivity for detection increases with ^{123}I-MIBG. For the detection of paragangliomas with ^{131}I-MIBG and ^{111}In–pentetreotide (Fig. 4.4) the sensitivity is 89% and 97% respectively[8] (Table 4.2). However, with ^{111}In-pentetreotide the relatively high activity in the kidneys is a drawback and limits the ability of this technique to identify small adrenal lesions.

NEUROBLASTOMA

Neuroblastoma is one of the common paediatric malignancies. The tumours arise from the primordial neural crest cells and are found in a variety of locations. Neuroblastoma may arise anywhere along the sympathetic chain, from the neck to the pelvis. It is a tumour that may spontaneously regress, rapidly progress and metastasize or cyto-differentiate into a benign ganglioneuroma. The majority of patients have an abdominal primary (65%) at presentation[9], more commonly adrenal in location. Neuroblastoma may metastasize early and may be disseminated to the liver, bone, bone marrow, lymph nodes and other organs.

Generally diagnosis is not a problem in these patients. However, to prognosticate, resectability of the lesion, DNA content, stage of disease, N-myc content and histological grade of the tumour are all important factors which need to be considered. At present two staging systems are used. The Paediatric Oncology Group system is based on tumour resectability and lymph node involvement, whereas the Evans' system uses tumour size and resectability, extension across the midline and presence of metastasis. Cross–sectional morphological imaging (CT or MRI) and skeletal scintigraphy

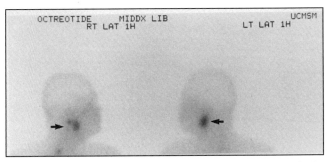

Fig. 4.4 A patient with bilateral glomus tumours (arrows) imaged 1 h after an intravenous injection of ^{111}In-pentetreotide

will accurately stage at least 95% of patients with thoraco-abdominal disease using Evans' classification[11]. CT is the best initial imaging modality to evaluate the extent of the disease and should be performed for every patient to determine the location and extent of the primary and metastatic lesions.

^{123}I-MIBG scintigraphy has been widely used for imaging patients with neuroblastoma. The sensitivity of MIBG for detecting this tumour is around 90%[8,12]. The main clinical indications are for the detection, staging and follow-up of this disease. The primary tumour, as well as soft tissue and bone marrow spread, may be detected, while the skeletal metastases can be assessed with conventional ^{99m}Tc-MDP bone scan[6]. Furthermore, where the tumour and its metastases are ^{123}I-MIBG avid, therapy with ^{131}I-MIBG can be used (Fig 4.5). ^{123}I-MIBG has the ability to detect early tumoral deposits in the bone marrow before osseous invasion occurs and with greater sensitivity than bone marrow biopsy. The reported cumulative sensitivity of MIBG scintigraphy was 92% and the specificity 100% in 779 children with neuroblastoma[8]. ^{111}In-pentetreotide has also been used for imaging these tumours; however, the reported sensitivity was 77%, which is lower than with ^{123}I-MIBG[8].

CARCINOID

Carcinoids are neuroendocrine tumours and are believed to arise from the enterochromaffin cells which are scattered throughout the body but occur primarily in the submucosa of the intestine

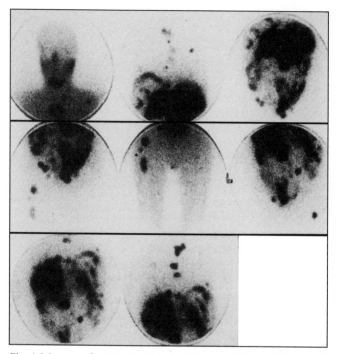

Fig. 4.5 *Images of a patient with neuroblastoma 18 h post injection of* [123]*I-MIBG. Top line: posterior views of the skull, chest and upper abdomen; middle line: posterior views of the lower abdomen and thighs, and anterior view of the lower abdomen; bottom line: anterior views of the upper abdomen and chest. Widespread extensive focal uptake is seen in metastases throughout the body. Such high uptake indicates that therapeutic benefit from* [131]*I-MIBG is likely*

and main bronchi. These tumours may produce 5–hydroxytryptamine or 5-hydroxytryptophan. The primary tumour is usually small, however, metastases which frequently occur in the liver, lymph nodes, peritoneum, lung and bones, are fairly large. Only in 10-40% of patients do symptoms occur. Metastases are present in 30-40% of patients at the time of initial detection, the regional lymph nodes being the most frequently involved. Radiolabelled MIBG concentrates in approximately 71% of these tumours. Carcinoids of midgut origin show a greater affinity for MIBG compared to those of hind- and foregut origin (Fig. 4.3).

The main indication for diagnostic ^{123}I-MIBG is to evaluate these patients for possible palliative therapy with ^{131}I-MIBG. Scintigraphy may be used to monitor the response to therapy.

ADRENAL CORTICAL TUMOURS

Radionuclide studies can also be used to characterise adrenal cortical tumours. The radiopharmaceuticals used most frequently to image adrenal cortical tumours are [131]I 6-ß-iodomethyl-19-norcholesterol (NP59) (dose 37 MBq [1 mCi]) and Selenium-75, [75]Se 6ß-selenomethyl-19-norcholesterol (dose 8 MBq), both of which concentrate in the adrenal tissue secreting steroid hormones.

The main clinical indication for this imaging test is in patients who have an incidentally discovered adrenal mass on CT and no evidence of excessive hormone secretion. Concentration of ^{131}I–NP59 or [75]Se-6ß-selenomethyl-19-norcholesterol within the lesion supports benignity. Unilateral decrease in tracer accumulation is not specific and may be associated with a variety of space-occupying lesions including metastases, adrenal carcinoma, cyst, haematoma and myelolipoma[13,14]. Depending on the patient population examined, 25-60% of these non-functioning lesions will prove to be adrenal metastases[15,16]. In these cases further investigation of the mass and underlying primary would be warranted. Other indications include localisation of an adenoma or demonstrate bilateral hyperplasia after a positive diagnosis has been made of Conn's or Cushing's syndrome.

More recently, ^{18}F-FDG PET imaging has also been used to characterise adrenal masses in cancer patients[17]. PET correctly differentiated benign from malignant lesions in these patients, thus obviating the need for percutaneous biopsy.

References

1. Shapiro B, Copp JE, Sisson JC, Eyre PL, Wallis J, Beierwaltes H. Iodine-131 metaiodobenzylguanidine for the locating of suspected phaeochromocytoma: experience in 400 cases. *J. of Nuclear Medicine* 1985; **26**: 576-585.

2. Hoefnagel CA. Radionuclide therapy revisited. *European J. of Nuclear Medicine* 1991; **18**: 408-413.

3. Lamberts SWJ, Krenning EP, Reubi JC. The role of somatostatin and its analogs in the diagnosis and treatment of tumours. *Endocrine Reviews* 1991; **12**: 450-482.

4. Bomanji J, Conry BG, Britton KE, Reznek RH. Imaging neural crest tumours with I-123 metaiodobenzylguanidine and x-ray computed tomography: a comparative study. *Clinical Radiology* 1988; **39**: 502-506.

5. Hanson MW, Feldman JM, Blinder RA, Moore JO, Coleman, R.E. Carcinoid tumour: Iodine-131 MIBG scintigraphy. *Radiology* 1989; **172**: 699-703.

6. Gordon I, Peters AM, Gutman A, Dicks-Mireaux C, Pritchard J. Skeletal assessment in neuroblastoma. The pitfalls of iodine-123 MIBG scans. *J. of Nuclear Medicine* 1990; **31**: 129-134.

7. Solanki KK, Bomanji J, Moyes J et al. A pharmacological guide to medicines which interfere with the biodistribution of radiolabelled meta-iodobenzylguanidine (MIBG). *Nuclear Medicine Comms* 1992; **13**: 513-521.

8. Hoefnagel CA. MIBG and somatostatin in oncology: role in the management of neural crest tumours. *European J. of Nuclear Medicine* 1994; **21**: 561-581.

9. Bousvaros A, Kirks DR, Grossman H. Imaging of neuroblastoma: A review. *Pediatric Radiology* 1986; **16**: 89.

10. Brodeur GM, Castleberry RP. Neuroblastoma. In : Pizzo P, Poplack DG eds. Principles and practice of pediatric oncology. 2nd ed. Philadelphia: *JB Lippincott*, 1993.11. Sotelo-Avila C, Gonzalez-Crussi F, Fowler JW. Complete and incomplete forms of Beckwith-Wiedemann syndrome: Their oncogenic potential. *J. of Pediatrics* 1980; **96**: 47-50.

12. Troncone L, Rufini V, Montemaggi M, Danza F.M, Lasorella A, Mastrangelo R. The diagnostic and therapeutic utility radioiodinated metaiodobenzylguanidine (MIBG). 5 years' experience. *European J. of Nuclear Medicine* 1990; **16**: 325-335.

13. Francis IR, Smid A, Gross MD, et al. Adrenal masses in oncologic patients. Functional and morphologic evaluation. *Radiology* 1988; **166**: 353-356.

14. Gross MD, Shapiro B, Bouffard AJ, et al. Distinguishing benign from malignant euadrenal masses. *Annals of Internal Medicine* 1988; **109**: 613-618.

15. Abecassis M, McLoughlin M, Langer B, Kudlow JE. Serendipitous adrenal masses: prevalence, significance, and management. *American J. of Surgery* 1985; **149**: 783-788.

16. Khafagi F, Gross MD, Shapiro B et al. Clinical significance of the large adrenal mass. *Brit. J. of Surgery* 1991; **78**: 828-833.

17. Boland GW, Goldberg MA, Lee MJ et al. Indeterminate adrenal mass in patients with cancer: Evaluation at PET with 2-[F-18]-fluoro-2-deoxy-d-glucose. *Radiology* 1995; **194**: 131-134.

Gastroendocrine Tumours

INTRODUCTION

Endocrine tumours of the pancreas and bowel can secrete several hormones, each with varying degrees of biological activity. Generally patients with these tumours present with various clinical features and syndromes. Despite the availability of several imaging techniques, the localisation of these tumours remains difficult for the endocrinologist, radiologist and nuclear medicine physician. Recently several new modalities such as magnetic resonance imaging (MRI), arterial stimulation sampling and receptor scintigraphy have been developed.

SOMATOSTATIN RECEPTOR SCINTIGRAPHY

^{111}In-[DTPA-D-Phe^1]-octreotide (^{111}In-pentetreotide)

In recent years somatostatin has emerged as a major regulatory neuropeptide with multiple biological actions. Somatostatin receptors have been demonstrated in tumours of the central nervous system, breast, lung and lymphoid tissue and in most neuroendocrine neoplasms. The presence of these receptors on the tumours provides the possibility of imaging them with radiolabelled somatostatin analogues (^{123}I-labelled Tyr^3-octreotide and ^{111}In-[DTPA-D-Phe^1]-octreotide). Between 80 and 120 MBq (2.1-3.2 mCi) of ^{111}In-[DTPA-D-Phe^1]-octreotide (^{111}In-pentetreotide) is injected intravenously and images of the whole body (anterior and posterior) are acquired at 1 h, 4 h and 24 h. Patients need to be off octreotide therapy.

Tumour type	% Scans positive	Tumour type	% Scans positive
GASTROENDOCRINE TUMOURS			
Gastrinomas	80%	Insulinomas	61%
Glucagonomas	95%	Somatostatinomas	100%
Carcinoid	86%	VIPomas	80%
OTHER TUMOURS			
Breast ca.	74%	Lymphomas (H)	83%
		(NH)	35%
Small cell lung ca.	95%	Meningiomas	100%
Neuroblastomas	77%	Medullary carcinoma of thyroid	66%
Pituitary adenomas	68%		
NH = Non-Hodgkin's; H = Hodgkin's			

Table 5.1 *Frequency of positive scans according to tumour type using* ^{111}*In-pentetreotide*

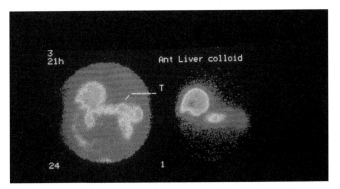

Fig. 5.1 *Patient with an insulinoma. Images were acquired with* ^{111}*In–pentetreotide. The left images in anterior projection show the tumour T. The right image shows the liver outline on a conventional liver* ^{99m}*Tc colloid scan*

37

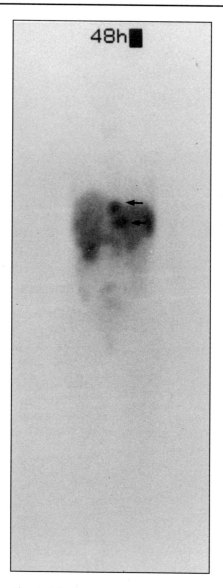

Fig. 5.2 *Anterior whole-body image of a patient with a metastatic gastrinoma. Focal and increased tracer uptake is seen in the liver metastases (arrows)*

Scintigraphic data from more than 1200 patients collected from multiple centres[1,2,3,4,5,6] are summarised in Table 5.1. A wide range in the percentage of positive scans was noted, depending on the receptor status, type of tumour imaged and number of patients evaluated. The main advantage of radiolabelled somatostatin scintigraphy is its ability to image the whole body and detect tumours or their metastases as small as 1 cm, especially in areas not under clinical suspicion. Secondly, this technique can be used to monitor the effects of chemotherapy in these patients[2]. Thirdly, positive uptake may predict successful therapy with octreotide medication in relieving symptoms.

Islet Cell Tumours

Insulinomas (Fig. 5.1), gastrinomas (Fig 5.2), glucagonomas, somatostatinomas and other functioning tumours are generally visualised with ^{111}In-pentetreotide scintigraphy. None of these neoplasms show any avidity for ^{123}I-MIBG. For imaging these tumours scintigraphy should not be the first line of investigation. However, imaging is extremely useful in patients with equivocal lesions on CT, or a negative CT in a patient with biochemical evidence of a functioning tumour.

PANCREATIC CARCINOMAS

CT is the mainstay for the diagnosis and staging of pancreatic carcinoma. However, it has difficulties in differentiating these tumours from mass-forming pancreatitis. In this context ^{18}F–FDG is useful. Stollufuss et al.[7] evaluated 76 patients with known pancreatic mass and showed that PET had a sensitivity of 96% and a specificity of 87%, while CT gave a sensitivity of 72% and a specificity of 81%. However, caution should be exercised as inflammatory tissue might also show some degree of uptake.

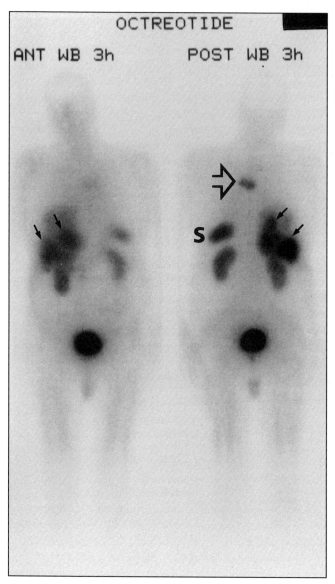

Fig. 5.3 ^{111}*In-pentetreotide scans of a patient with metastatic carcinoid tumour. Small arrows indicate metastases in liver. Open arrow shows a metastatic lesion in T5.*
S = normal tracer uptake in spleen

CARCINOID

[111]In-pentetreotide has also been used for imaging patients with carcinoid tumours (Fig 5.3). The cumulative sensitivity of detection for ^{111}In-pentetreotide is 86%. In comparison ^{123}I–MIBG scintigraphy has a cumulative sensitivity of 71%[8]. From a diagnostic point of view ^{111}In-pentetreotide is the initial procedure of choice in these patients. ^{111}In-pentetreotide scintigraphy can also be used as a predictor of response to palliative therapy.

VASOACTIVE INTESTINAL PEPTIDE-RECEPTOR IMAGING

More recently radioiodinated vasoactive intestinal peptide has been used for imaging intestinal adenocarcinomas and various endocrine tumours which express a large number of high-affinity receptors for vasoactive intestinal peptide (VIP). Seventy nine patients were imaged. ^{123}I-labelled synthetic VIP, a 28-amino-acid neuroendocrine mediator was used for imaging[9]. Initial imaging results were encouraging, but further studies are necessary to clarify the role of this technique.

References

1. Lamberts SWJ, Krenning EP, Reubi JC. The role of somatostatin and its analogs in the diagnosis and treatment of tumours. *Endocrine Reviews* 1991; **12**: 450-482.

2. Krenning EP, Kwekkeboom DJ, Bakker WH, et al. Somatostatin receptor scintigraphy with ^{111}In-DTPA-D-Phe[1] and ^{123}I-Tyr[3]-octreotide: Rotterdam experience with more than 1000 patients. *European J. of Nuclear Medicine* 1993; **20**: 716-731.

3. Ur E, Bomanji J, Mather S et al. Localisation of neuroendocrine tumours and insulinomas using radiolabelled somatostatin analogues, ^{123}I-Tyr-[3]-octreotide and ^{111}In-pentetreotide. *Clinical Endocrinology* 1993; **38**: 501-506.

4. Bomanji J, Ur E, Mather S et al. A scintigraphic comparison of I-123 metaiodobenzylguanidine (MIBG) and I-123 labelled somatostatin analogue (Tyr-3-octreotide) in metastatic carcinoid tumours. *J. of Nuclear Medicine* 1992; **33**: 1121-1124

5. King CMP, Reznek RH, Bomanji J, et al. Imaging neuroendocrine tumours with radiolabelled somatostatin analogues and x-ray computed tomography: a comparative study. *Clinical Radiology* 1993; **48**: 386-391.

6. Lipp RW, Silly H, Ranner G et al. Radiolabelled octreotide for the demonstration of somatostatin receptors in malignant lymphoma and lymphadenopathy. *J. of Nuclear Medicine* 1995; **36**: 13-18.

7. Stollufuss JC, Schonberger JA, Fries H, Beger HG, Reske SN. Improved diagnosis of pancreatic carcinoma with FDG-PET compared to CT in non-invasive imaging modalities. *European J. of Nuclear Medicine* 1994; **21**: 759.

8. Hoefnagel CA. MIBG and somatostatin in oncology: role in the management of neural crest tumours. *European J. of Nuclear Medicine* 1994; **21**: 561-581.

9. Virgolini I, Raderer M, Kurtaran A et al. Vasoactive intestinal peptide-receptor imaging for the localization of intestinal adenocarcinomas and endocrine tumours. *New England J. of Medicine* 1994; **331**: 1116-1121.

Lung Cancer

INTRODUCTION

Lung cancer is a major cause of death and disability throughout the world and is the commonest malignant disease in Western Europe.

The evaluation of the patient with suspected lung cancer remains a difficult clinical problem even though multiple imaging techniques are available. To determine malignancy in a single pulmonary nodule and to stage lung cancer still requires a biopsy in most patients. Stage of the disease and tumour cell type are the two most important determinants of treatment and prognosis. For practical purposes the disease can be divided into small-cell lung carcinoma (SCLC) and non-small-cell lung carcinoma (NSCLC).

Investigations

In virtually all patients considered for curative treatment of lung cancer, imaging is required to evaluate the extent of disease. The main indications for imaging are to detect hilar, mediastinal, chest wall and extrathoracic metastases. Detection of hilar, mediastinal or chest wall involvement eliminates thoracotomy or surgical excision, since the probability of disease-free survival is less than 10% at 5 years in these patients. This question is of substantial importance in NSCLC, where cure is generally possible only with complete excision of viable tumour from thorax. The most accurate method of pre-thoracotomy assessment of N2 (ipsilateral mediastinal node involvement) and N3 (contralateral or supraclavicular node involvement) disease is mediastinoscopy. However, it is a significant surgical procedure and a small percentage of mediastinal lesions may be missed. Chest x-ray remains the most cost-effective screening and diagnostic procedure. However, it cannot be relied on to select patients for mediastinoscopy. CT scans play an important role in assessing spread to mediastinum undetected on planar x-rays. CT has a sensitivity of 95% and a specificity of 80% in predicting mediastinal metastases and has been recommended as the imaging modality of choice for central lesions. Many centres currently use CT of the mediastinum as a screening examination, opting for mediastinoscopy in those patients with enlarged mediastinal nodes on CT. In other words patients with a normal CT result can proceed directly to thoracotomy because even if their nodes are involved they are easy to resect and the prognosis remains relatively good. Routine MRI of all lung cancers remains unnecessary and should be reserved for cases where local tumour invasion of mediastinum and paravertebral regions on CT is unclear. Both CT and MRI imaging may miss up to 40% of mediastinal lymph node metastases when compared to surgical staging[1,2]. Furthermore, differentiation of residual or recurrent disease and post-surgical or post-radiation fibrosis with these morphological imaging modalities is poor.

Gallium-67/Thallium-201

Nuclear medicine techniques address some of these problems and provide functional information on the tumour and its metastases in a non-invasive fashion and help to refine further the follow-up and management of the patient[3]. In this context both ^{201}Tl and ^{67}Ga have been evaluated extensively (Fig 6.1; Fig 6.2). Tracer uptake is generally higher in anaplastic and epidermoid tumours and lower in adenocarcinoma. There is good correlation between ^{67}Ga uptake and the change in tumour size after treatment as determined radiographically. After therapy, serial ^{67}Ga scans may demonstrate metastatic lesions long before these become visible radiographically. Richardson et al[4] prospectively evaluated CT, ^{67}Ga and surgical sampling of mediastinal tissue in patients with bronchogenic carcinoma. [67]Ga scanning gave a sensitivity of 55% and CT 61% while the specificity was 96% and 81% respectively. In a second study of 113 patients, CT and ^{201}Tl scintigraphy were compared. It was shown that the sensitivity

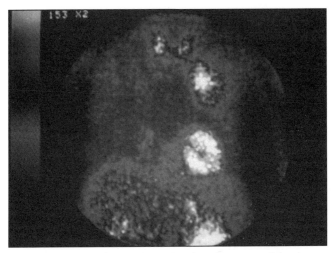

Fig. 6.1 *Bronchial carcinoma imaged with* ^{201}*Tl. Anterior chest view. Uptake can be seen in the thyroid, heart, liver and spleen, and a focal area of uptake in the left chest is due to a bronchial carcinoma. (Courtesy of Professor J. McKillop)*

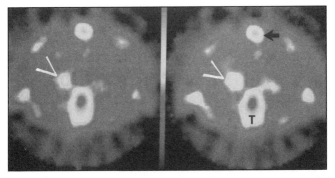

Fig. 6.2 ^{67}*Ga scan in a patient with an adenocarcinoma in the right hilum. SPET images (transaxial slices) show abnormal focal uptake (arrowhead) corresponding to the tumour in the hilar region. Normal tracer uptake is noted in the sternum (arrow) and thoracic vertebrae (T)*

and specificity of CT for detecting cancerous nodes were 62%
and 80% respectively, while the figures for ^{201}Tl were 76%
and 92% respectively. ^{201}Tl did not result in a substantial
increase in accuracy in patients with normal-sized lymph
nodes at CT[5]. It was suggested that instead of
mediastinoscopy, ^{201}Tl scintigraphy should be performed in all
patients with enlarged lymph nodes.

It should be noted that scintigraphy, although useful in
identifying extrathoracic disease from NSCLC, fails
specifically in the brain and osseous tissues. Bone scintigraphy
remains one of the most sensitive and cost-effective techniques
to detect bone metastases from lung cancer, especially in
clinical stage III disease if considering curative therapy.
This has been discussed elsewhere[6]. Detection of soft tissue
lesions requires other scintigraphic imaging techniques.

RADIOLABELLED MONOCLONAL ANTIBODIES

Besides ^{67}Ga and ^{201}Tl, other more sensitive and specific
scintigraphic imaging techniques are now becoming available.
Recently, radiolabelled monoclonal antibodies (MoAb) have
been used for imaging NSCLC and SCLC[7,8]. In a phase III
multicentre trial for staging SCLC using Fab fragment of
MoAb NR-LU-10 labelled with ^{99m}Tc, 96 patients were
evaluated[8,9]. Staging with MoAb was compared with staging
using a standard battery of tests. Radioimmunoscintigraphy
(RIS) had a positive predictive value of 95-100% compared
with 96-100% for the standard battery of tests combined.
None of the other diagnostic tests on their own was as
sensitive or accurate as RIS. In 15% of patients who were
thought to have limited disease, RIS upstaged the diagnosis to
extensive disease, which was subsequently corroborated with
other imaging modalities. The study concluded that if RIS
showed extensive disease, the positive predictive value was so
high that no further tests were required. On the other hand if
only limited disease was outlined then further standard tests
might be helpful to detect 10% of the patients who had occult
spread. Of particular interest was the detection of unsuspected
bone marrow involvement in the absence of bony lesions on

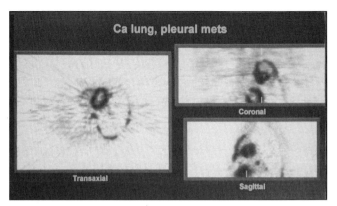

Figure 6.3 *Adenocarcinoma of left lung with pleural metastases.*
¹⁸F-FDG PET study showed a hypermetabolic focus localised to the
hilar region with pleural involvement of the left lung

bone scintigraphy or positive histological results on bone
marrow aspirates.

Several investigators have reported on the results of ^{99m}Tc NR-
LU-10 Fab imaging in patients with NSCLC[7,10]. Primary lung
lesions and diseased nodes have been imaged with a sensitivity
of 94% and 95% respectively. The sensitivity of CT in
assessment of nodal metastases was 81-88%. Detection rates for
RIS were 91-100% for all organs except bones, where the
detection rate was 25%. It is quite clear that RIS is useful in
NSCLC patients to delineate lesions, especially where CT
imaging identifies nodes which are slightly enlarged or look
suspicious (nodes less than 1-1.5 cm in diameter in different
series were considered normal).

¹⁸F-FLUORODEOXYGLUCOSE (¹⁸F-FDG) PET IMAGING

¹⁸F-FDG PET scintigraphy has been performed in patients with
lung cancer[11,12,13] (Fig 6.3). Preliminary studies have shown a
high sensitivity, specificity and accuracy for evaluating
radiologically indeterminate solitary pulmonary nodules.
¹⁸F–FDG has a sensitivity of 83% and a specificity of 90% in
differentiating malignant from benign nodules. Malignant
nodules have increased uptake while benign nodules have

minimal uptake. Abnormal ^{18}F-FDG accumulation has also been noted in involved nodes irrespective of the nodal size. However, caution should be exercised as granulomatous diseases such as sarcoid and tuberculosis show high uptake of ^{18}F FDG. ^{18}F-FDG PET studies have also been shown to be accurate in staging lung tumours and for differentiating between scar and residual tumour. Gupta et al[14] correctly predicted presence or absence of tumour in 19 patients previously treated for lung malignancy. Similar results have been reported by others[15].

^{111}IN-[DTPA-D-PHE^1]-OCTREOTIDE (^{111}IN-PENTETREOTIDE)

^{111}In-pentetreotide scintigraphy has also been used for imaging SCLC and NSCLC[16,17]. In the two studies the sensitivity of detecting the primary lesion was high (>95%), however, for metastatic disease reported sensitivity was 45% and 50% respectively. Overall, the number of patients evaluated was small and the sensitivity for detecting metastatic disease is fairly low to justify use of this radiopharmaceutical at this stage.

PREOPERATIVE FUNCTIONAL LUNG ASSESSMENT

Less frequently, lung scintigraphy has been used for preoperative functional assessment of lung cancer patients scheduled to undergo pulmonary resection. In these cases scintigraphy can be used to predict postoperative lung function and postoperative mortality. Wernly et al.[18], in a study on 85 patients, found that the product of preoperative forced expiratory volume in the first second (FEV1) and percentage scintigraphic perfusion (or xenon-133 ventilation) was a good predictor of postoperative FEV1. Other investigators have shown that a predicted postoperative FEV1 of 0.8-1.0 L, estimated by quantitative pulmonary scintigraphy, yields an acceptable (15%) postoperative mortality[19]. In a further prospective study of 55 consecutive patients with suspected malignant lesions of the lung[20], a predicted postoperative FEV1 of 40% or more of the predicted value (based on preoperative spirometric and pulmonary scintigraphic measurements) was associated with no postoperative mortality in 47 patients, whereas a value of less than 40% of the predicted amount was associated with 50% mortality (three of six patients).

References

1. Webb WR, Gatsonis C, Zerhouni EA, et al. CT and MRI imaging in staging non-small cell bronchogenic carcinoma: report of the Radiologic Diagnostic Oncology Group. *Radiology* 1991; **178**: 705-713.

2. McLoud TC, Bourgouin PM, Greenberg RW et al. Bronchogenic carcinoma: analysis of staging in the mediastinum with CT by correlative lymph node mapping and sampling. *Radiology* 1992; **182**: 319-323.

3. Abdel-Dayem HM, Scott A, Macapinlac H, Larson S. Tumour imaging in lung cancer. *European J. of Nuclear Medicine* 1994; **21**: 57-81.

4. Richardson JV, Zenk BA, Rossi NP et al. Preoperative non-invasive mediastinal staging in bronchogenic carcinoma. *Surgery* 1980; **88**: 382.

5. Yokoi K, Okuyama A, Mori K et al. Mediastinal lymph node metastases from lung cancer: evaluation with Tl-201 SPECT-Comparison with CT. *Radiology* 1994; **192**: 813–817.

6. McKillop JH, Fogelman I. Oncology. In, Benign and malignant bone disease. Churchill Livingstone, London 1991; 30-52.

7. Friedman S, Sullivan K, Salk D et al. Staging non-small cell carcinoma of the lung using technetium-99m-labelled monoclonal antibodies. *Hematolo. Oncol. Clin. North America* 1991; **4**: 1069-1078

8. Nelp WB, Griep RG, Salk D et al. Staging of small cell cancer of the lung using Tc-99m labelled antibody (Fab). In: Haseman MK, ed. Frontiers of nuclear medicine: diagnostic uses of radiolabelled monoclonal antibodies. Washington, DC. *American College of Nuclear Physicians* 1992; 15-20.

9. Abrams P, Fer M, Fabion C et al. A new procedure for staging small cell lung cancer (SCLC): gamma camera imaging using a technetium-99m labelled monoclonal antibody Fab. *Am. Soc. Clin. Oncol.* 1990; **9**: A895.

10. Rusch V, Macapinlac H, Heelman R et al. Nr-LU-10

monoclonal antibody scanning: a helpful new adjunct to CT in evaluating non-small cell lung cancer. *J. Thorac. Cardiovas. Surg.* 1993; **106**: 200-204.

11. Kubota K, Matsuzawa T, Fujiwara T et al. Differential diagnosis of lung tumour with positron emmission tomography: a prospective study. *J. of Nuclear Medicine* 1990; **31**: 1927-1933.

12. Strauss LG, Conti PS. The application of PET in clinical oncology. *J. of Nuclear Medicine* 1991; **32**: 623-648.

13. Gupta NC, Frank AR, Dewan NA et al. Solitary pulmonary nodules: detection of malignancy with PET with 2-[F-18] fluoro-2-deoxy glucose. *Radiology* 1992; **184**: 441-444.

14. Gupta NC, Dewan NA, Frank AR, Millard J, Scott W. Presurgical evaluation of patients with suspected malignant solitary pulmonary nodules (SPN) using PET-FDG imaging. *J. of Nuclear Medicine* 1993; **34**: 20P.

15. Inoue T, Kim EE, Komaki R et al. Detecting recurrent or residual lung cancer with FDG-PET. *J. Nuclear Medicine*, 1995 **36**:788-793

16. Kirsch CM, von Pawel J, Grau I, Tatsch K. Indium-111 pentetreotide in the diagnostic work-up of patients with bronchogenic carcinoma. *European J. of Nuclear Medicine* 1994; **21**: 1318-1325.

17. O'Byrne KJ, Ennis JT, Freyne PJ, Clancy LJ, Prichard JS, Carney DN. Scintigraphic imaging of small-cell lung cancer with [indium-111] pentetreotide, a radiolabelled somatostatin analogue. *British J. of Cancer* 1994; **69**: 762-766.

18. Wernley JA, DeMeester TR, Kirchner PT et al. Clinical value of quantitative ventilation-perfusion lung scan in the surgical management of bronchogenic carcinoma. *J. of Thoracic and Cardiovascular Surgery* 1980; **80**: 535-543.

19. Boyesn PG, Block AJ, Olsen GN, Moulder PV, Harris JO, Ratwitscher RE. Prospective evaluation for pneumonectomy using the technetium-99m quantitative perfusion lung scan. *Chest* 1977; **72**: 422-425.

20. Markos J, Mullan BP, Hillman DR et al. Preoperative assessment as a predictor of mortality and morbidity after lung resection. *Am. Rev. Respir. Dis.* 1989; **139**: 902-910.

Abdominal and Pelvic Cancers

INTRODUCTION

The application of nuclear medicine to the management of patients with cancers of the gastrointestinal tract is becoming increasingly important. The general agents gallium-67, thallium-201 and ^{99m}Tc-MIBI have no consistent value for tumour imaging here. PET with ^{18}F-FDG is able to distinguish pancreatic cancer from chronic inactive pancreatitis and is being explored in recurrent colorectal cancer, neuroblastoma and lymphoma as an adjunct to CT and MRI imaging. The main radiolabelled agents for cancer management (excluding neural crest tumours and lymphomas described previously) are radiolabelled peptides and radiolabelled antibodies. Liver tumours are considered in the chapter titled 'Other tumours'. Colorectal, ovarian and prostate cancer will be considered here.

COLORECTAL CANCER

Primary colorectal cancer is the second most common neoplasm in men and the third most common in women. Primary diagnosis is by digital rectal examination, sigmoidoscopy, colonoscopy or double contrast barium enema. Flexible sigmoidoscopy is being introduced as a screening test. Radionuclide imaging has a small role in primary cancer. It may be used to detect a second unexpected primary tumour [1,2] or liver metastases. The main uses are in the detection of recurrent disease (Fig. 7.1) before and when serum markers such as CEA are elevated, in finding disease that is not radiologically evident, and in the demonstration that a mass seen radiologically contains viable tumour and is not just due to postsurgical fibrosis. The use of the

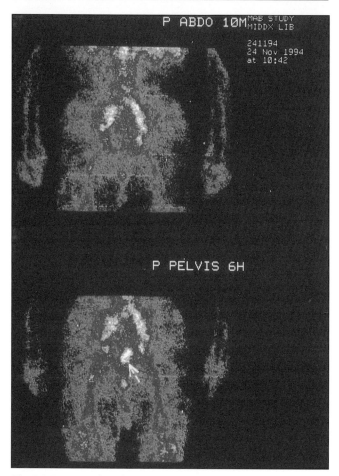

Fig. 7.1 *Patient with Dukes' C stage primary tumour 16 months after potentially curative therapy and borderline raised CEA levels. For imaging ^{99m}Tc-PR1A3, a monoclonal antibody reacting with colorectal cancer, was used. Upper panel: posterior pelvic view 10 min postinjection, showing activity in the iliac vessels. Lower panel: delayed view 6 h postinjection; arrow indicates the site of recurrence. The 10-min image acts as a template with which to compare the late 6-h image*

interoperative probe with radiolabelled antibodies has a place in determining that the tumour bed and the bowel for an anastomosis is free of disease, and that there are no involved lymph nodes outside the incision field[3].

The mechanism for imaging such tumours is by the use of radiolabelled antibodies which bind to the colorectal cancer cells (radioimmunoscintigraphy, RIS). Three types of antibody are used: one against the primitive antigen, carcinoembryonic antigen (CEA), which is used as a serum marker; one produced by using tumour extracts for immunisation of the mouse for development of the monoclonal antibody, such as B72.3 against TAG-72, a tumour-associated antigen which is partly shed; and one against that part of the complex molecule which releases CEA but which stays bound to the cancer cell membrane and is not shed, called PR1A3. ^{111}In-B72.3 is commercially available as Oncoscint (Cytogen) for imaging colorectal cancer[4,5], but the antigen with which it reacts is not expressed in about 20% of colorectal cancers. [99m]Tc anti-CEA is available as BW431/26 (Behring)[1,6].

The staging of colorectal cancer cannot be performed by using radiolabelled monoclonal antibodies against CEA, since CEA is trapped by normal nodes more effectively than by involved nodes. This is because once the carcinoma has broken through the basement membrane, the shed antigen travels in the local lymphatics and is held by the sinusoid lining cells of the lymph nodes. This is one of the disadvantages of using an antibody against an antigen that is shed. B72.3 also appears to have this problem[7] but PR1A3 does not[8].

Primary colorectal tumours are classified using the Dukes' staging and this is related to prognosis: the 5-year survival rates are 90% for Dukes' A, 60% for Dukes' B, and 30% for Dukes' C. Dukes' C is the commonest stage found at primary surgery and means that local lymph nodes are involved in the surgical specimen. There is a 50% chance of its recurrence at 1 year. Conventionally serial serum CEA is used to follow up such patients, but the non-specific rises and falls in serum CEA require that there is an increasing serum level during 3 successive months. RIS is being performed at the 1-year routine

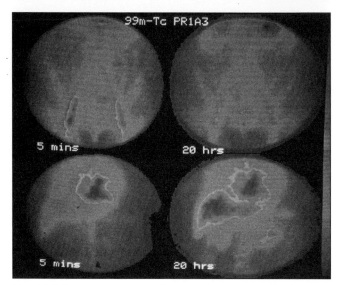

Fig. 7.2 *Colon cancer images with* ^{99m}*Tc-PR1A3, a monoclonal antibody reacting with colorectal cancer. Left: images at 5 min of the pelvis and abdomen show high blood pool in the heart and iliac vessels. Right: images at 20 h show some activity in the kidneys and bladder (top right) and a focal area of increased uptake in the splenic flexure inferior and to the right of the liver and cardiac blood pool activity (bottom right). Non-specific uptake decreases with time while specific uptake in colorectal cancer increases with time. The early image acts as the template with which to compare the later image at 20 h. (Courtesy of Dr. M. Granowska)*

follow-up appointment after primary surgery and Dukes' C staging. Already up to 30% of patients have clearly demonstrated recurrent disease at a time when their serum CEA was still within the normal range[9]. Such early disease detection was confirmed and led to the initiation of treatment (either second surgery or radiotherapy) an opportunity that would have been missed if reliance had been placed only on the serum CEA and symptoms during follow-up. This type of finding gives a reminder that the tumour has to be of an adequate size to release a sufficient load of CEA to raise the serum level above normal whereas RIS gives a direct evaluation of the presence of a recurrence as well as locating its sites. Once serum CEA is elevated, then RIS with an anti–CEA or other anti-colorectal cancer antibody is able to locate the site of the tumour at a time when conventional radiology may be negative. However, it must be remembered that inflammatory bowel diseases also release CEA, e.g. Crohn's disease. In such a case serial imaging shows no change in position of the bowel abnormality, whereas CEA released into intestinal contents changes in position on serial imaging.

In a recent survey of RIS in gastrointestinal tumours average sensitivity of 79%, specificity of 85% and accuracy of 81% was reported in more than 1700 patients using a battery of radiolabelled monoclonal antibodies and their fragments [1].

Excellent results are obtained using ^{99m}Tc-labelled antibodies, particularly PR1A3 (Fig 7.2). A great advantage is that the ^{99m}Tc label is available at all times whereas ^{111}In may take several days to order. ^{99m}Tc RIS is undertaken as follows. 600 MBq of ^{99m}Tc (16 mCi) on 0.5-1 mg of murine antibody is injected intravenously and anterior and posterior images of the upper and lower abdomen are taken at 10 min, together with a squat view of the pelvis. The frequency of clinical reactions is of the order of 1:1000, being similar to that for bone scans. Further images are taken at 6-8 h together with SPET of the pelvis and again at 20–24 h. If the probe is to be used, this imaging should be arranged to terminate on the morning of surgery so the probe is used intra-abdominally at about 24-26 hours after the injection of the ^{99m}Tc-labelled monoclonal antibody.

For ^{111}In-labelled antibody, 150 MBq (4 mCi) is injected intravenously and images are taken at 10 min, 24 h and 72 h after injection. SPET is usually performed at 24 h. The absorbed radiation dose from ^{99m}Tc RIS is significantly lower than that of ^{111}In, yet the signal is three times greater. Because the metabolised fragments of the ^{99m}Tc-labelled antibody go to the kidney, the liver uptake is much reduced and positive uptake in liver metastases is much easier to see than when ^{111}In is used. There is also less bowel and marrow uptake of the ^{99m}Tc-labelled antibody as compared with ^{111}In–labelled antibody. The sensitivity and specificity are greater with the ^{99m}Tc label and it brings a technique to the routine Nuclear Medicine Department in a district hospital.

RIS is therefore earning an important place in the follow-up of patients after primary colorectal cancer surgery both in the early detection of recurrence, when serum markers are normal, or in localising it when they are elevated and in determining the viability of a radiologically detected mass.

Hepatic metastases represent a special problem in recurrent disease. Liver metastases can take on four appearances. First a large defect on the 5 min image may persist throughout the series of images and this may be due to other diagnoses. Secondly, a defect may appear on the 5-min image which gets smaller on the later images, perhaps with an area of increased uptake around its periphery. Thirdly, a defect on the 5-min image may disappear apparently into a normal image of the liver and lastly, a normal liver on the 5-min image may develop a focal area of increased uptake on the 22 h image[2].

Recently, radiolabelled peptides have also been used for colorectal imaging. The development of ^{123}I vasoactive intestinal peptide, VIP, as an imaging agent gives positive results in a number of colorectal cancers and also in gastric cancer including involvement of the Virchow node and in carcinoid tumours[10].

GYNAECOLOGICAL CANCER

Monoclonal antibodies used for targeting gynaecological cancer are of four main types. The first is anti-HCG against the oncofetal protein human chorio-gonadotrophic hormone, used to detect choriocarcinoma[11]. The second type of anticancer monoclonal antibody is one which reacts against a surface glycoprotein of normal cells that lie inside tubes, such as the milk ducts of the breast and the inner surface of an ovarian follicle. Such antigens are remote from the bloodstream so a monoclonal antibody against them will not normally react *in vivo*. However, the architectural disruption that every cancer causes, brings large quantities of such cell-bound antigens into contact with the blood, where they are detectable using RIS. HMFG1 and HMGF2 antibodies against the human milk fat globule surface lining protein of the milk duct and ovarian follicle, which are now called polymorphic

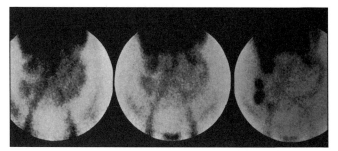

Fig. 7.3 *Ovarian cancer recurrence imaged with* ^{99m}Tc-SM3, *a monoclonal antibody reacting with ovarian and breast cancer. Images at 10 min (left), 6 h (centre) and 24 h (right). In the first image a halo of ascites can be seen with vascular activity; at 24 hours two focal areas in the right flank and one over the right iliac vessel are clearly evident. These are the local recurrences causing the malignant ascites. Liver and renal uptake is also evident. (Courtesy of Dr. M. Granowska)*

epithelial mucin (PEM) antibodies, are of this type and are very effective in detecting ovarian and endometrial cancer. SM3, stripped mucin antibody, is the latest version of this sort of agent; it has higher specificity for breast and ovarian cancer and a low reactivity with normal tissue and benign tumours[12]. The third type of monoclonal antibody is one against a cancer cell protein which is present in larger amounts than in normal cells. Such antibodies include anti-placental alkaline phosphatase (PLAP), which reacts with seminomas and ovarian cancers, OC-125, which is also used as a tumour marker, OVTL-3[13] and MOV-18[14]. The latter is against a surface protein concerned with folic acid metabolism. The fourth type of antibody is against a synthetic antigen such as 17OH-82. For imaging, such antibodies have been labelled with ^{123}I, ^{111}In or ^{99m}Tc. Initially provided as murine antibodies, they are now being developed as humanised antibodies so that they can be administered in larger amounts for therapy without inducing human anti-mouse antibody (HAMA) responses. The method of imaging is as for colorectal cancer.

There are two main clinical applications of monoclonal antibodies in gynaecological cancer. First, they may be used for the detection of recurrent ovarian cancer (Fig. 7.3), and in particular for assessing the effect of chemotherapy by means of RIS, thereby reducing the need for second-look laparotomy. Secondly, they may be used to determine whether a radiologically evident mass is due to recurrence or not, particularly in the pelvis. Ultrasound, because of the problems of bowel gas, and CT, because of the lack of definition of tissue planes, have difficulty in detecting recurrent disease in the pelvis. This is particularly so because ovarian cancer may recur as thin plaques which are well able to take up the antibody but are not easy to see using a physical technique. In a recent survey of RIS in ovarian cancer average sensitivity of 78%, specificity of 80% and accuracy of 77% was reported in more than 550 patients [1]. In a prospective study the sensitivity of RIS for the detection of ovarian cancer after chemotherapy exceeded 89%, compared with 34% for ultrasound, and 57% for x-ray CT[15]. RIS is also required to demonstrate specific uptake before the application of radiolabelled immunotherapy (RIT). Further areas of application are a) the detection of ovarian cancer before or when serum markers are elevated, b) the demonstration that an ultrasound-detected lesion in a well woman is likely to be malignant before primary surgery is undertaken and c) use in conjunction with the preoperative probe.

PROSTATE CANCER

Prostate cancer is the second most common cancer in men and appears to be increasing in prevalence. Small primary prostate cancer may be seen in the majority of people over 70 coming to post mortem and there is some controversy as to the need to perform primary prostate cancer surgery in the very old when cancer is detected. In the under 50s it accounts for less than 1% of cancers. The detection of cancer of the prostate either by digital rectal examination or by screening for the serum marker, prostate specific antigen (PSA), leads to primary surgery. This may be local or radical. The reason for radical surgery is related to prognosis. If a single lymph node is involved locally then the 5-year survival rate falls from about 85% to under 50%. It is therefore important to detect whether the prostate cancer has spread outside the capsule and/or is involving local nodes. MRI, CT and prostate RIS[16] are all being evaluated in this role.

The anti-prostate membrane antigen monoclonal antibody CYT-356, labelled with ^{111}In, and CYT-351, labelled with ^{99m}Tc, have been developed by Cytogen. Imaging protocol is as described for colorectal cancer but serial SPET at 6 h and 24 h is essential. Specific uptake of the antibody increases with time between these two images whereas blood and non-specific uptake decreases as in the genitalia. Comparison of serial SPET images enables detection of spread into local lymph nodes and spread of prostate cancer through the prostate capsule[17].

Seminomas are well detected by anti-placental alkaline phosphatase antibodies labelled with ^{123}I, ^{111}In or ^{99m}Tc, but the management of testicular cancer is by surgery and radiotherapy.

RADIOPEPTIDE IMAGING

[111]In-pentetreotide has been used for imaging small-cell cancers of the gastrointestinal tract and the gastroendocrine tumours: insulinoma, gastrinoma, VIPoma, glucagonoma etc.[18]. More recently ^{123}I-vasoactive intestinal peptide may also demonstrate carcinoids, colorectal, gastric and pancreatic cancers[10]. These are discussed in the Gastroendocrine Tumours section.

In conclusion RIS and radiopeptide scintigraphy are having an increasing role in the management of patients with abdominal cancer. The main limitations are the availability of the monoclonal antibodies and the costs of the radiopeptides, of ^{111}In and of the commercially available monoclonal antibodies.

References

1. Bischof Delaloye A, Delaloye B. Tumour imaging with monoclonal antibodies. *Seminars in Nuclear Medicine* 1995, **25**:144-164.

2. Granowska M, Britton KE, Mather SJ et al. Radioimmunoscintigraphy with technetium-99m labelled monoclonal antibody 1A3, in colorectal cancer. *European J. of Nuclear Medicine* 1993; **20**: 690-698.

3. Aprile C. Interoperative radioimmunolocalisation of colorectal cancer: a review. *Int. J. of Biological Markers* 1993; **8**: 166-171.

4. Muxi A, Pons F, Herranz R et al. Radioimmunoscintigraphy of colorectal carcinoma with a ^{111}In-labelled anti TAG-72 monoclonal antibody. *Nuclear Medicine Comms.* 1993; **14**: 775-787.

5. Kmiot WA, Stonelake P, Sagar G et al. Radioimmunoscintigraphy of recurrent colorectal carcinoma using ^{111}In-labelled murine monoclonal antibody B72.3: a comparison with contrast-enhanced computed tomography. *Nuclear Medicine Comms.* 1993; **14**: 788-791.

6. Muxi A, Sola M, Bassa P et al. Radioimmunoscintigraphy of colorectal carinoma with a ^{99m}Tc-labelled anti-CEA monoclonal antibody (BW 432/16). *Nuclear Medicine Comms.* 1993; **14**: 261-270.

7. Kuhn JA, Corbisiero RM, Buras RR et al. Interoperative gamma detection with presurgical imaging in colon cancer. *Archives of Surgery* 1991; **126**: 1398-1403.

8. Granowska M, Jass JB, Britton KE, Northover JMA. A prospective study of the use of the ^{111}In-labelled monoclonal antibody against carcinoembryonic antigen in colorectal cancer and of some biological factors affecting its uptake. *Int. J. of Colorectal Diseases* 1989; **4**: 97-108.

9. Abdel-Nabi H, Doerr RJ. Clinical applications of Indium-111-labelled monoclonal antibody imaging in colorectal cancer patients. *Seminar in Nuclear Medicine* 1993; **23**: 99-113.

10. Virgolini I, Raderer M, Kurtaran A et al. Vasoactive intestinal peptide-receptor imaging for the localization of intestinal adenocarcinomas and endocrine tumours. *New England J. of Medicine* 1994; **331**: 1116-1121.

11. Begent RHJ, Stanway G, Jones BE et al. Radioimmunolocalisation of tumours by external scintigraphy after administration of ^{131}I antibody to human gonadotrophin: preliminary communication. *J. of Royal Society of Medicine* 1980; **73**: 624-625.

12. Granowska M, Britton KE, Mather SJ et al.
    Radioimmunoscintigraphy with technetium-99m-labelled
    monocloncal antibody, SM3, in gynaecological cancer.
    European J. of Nuclear Medicine 1993b; **20**: 483-489.

13. Tibben JB, Massuger LFAG, Claessens RAMJ et al.
    Tumour detection and localization using ^{99m}Tc-labelled
    OV-TL-3Fab' in patients suspected of ovarian cancer.
    Nuclear Medicine Comms. 1992; **13**: 885-893.

14. Crippa F, Buraggi GL, DiRe E et al.
    Radioimmunoscintigraphy of ovarian cancer with the
    MOV-18 monoclonal antibody. *European J. of Cancer*
    1991; **27**: 724-729.

15. Peltier P, Wiharto K, Dutin J-P et al. Correlative imaging
    study in the diagnosis of ovarian cancer recurrences.
    European J. of Nuclear Medicine 1992; **19**: 1006-1010.

16. Textor JH, O'Neil CE. Current applications of
    immunoscintigraphy in prostate cancer. *J. of Nuclear
    Medicine* 1993; **34**: 549-553.

17. Chengazi VU, Feneley M, Granowska M et al.
    Radioimmunoscintigraphy of soft tissue recurrence of
    prostatic cancer with Tc-99m labelled monoclonal
    antibody. *European J. of Nuclear Medicine* 1994; **21**: 770.

18. Krenning EP, Kwekkeboom DJ, Bakker WH et al.
    Somatostatin receptor scintigraphy with ^{111}In-DTPA-D-Phe[1]
    and ^{123}I-Tyr3-octreotide: Rotterdam experience with more
    than 1000 patients. *European J. of Nuclear Medicine*
    1993; **20**: 716-731.

Breast Cancer

INTRODUCTION

Because breast cancer is so common there is controversy over its management. Radical mastectomy has been replaced by simpler operations, on the one hand to preserve as much breast tissue as possible and on the other to reduce the complications of an extended lymphadenectomy in the axilla. It is generally agreed that self-examination is not a reliable way of detecting early breast cancer and screening mammography is recommended. Although this screening is of value, radiologists can differ, sometimes substantially, in their interpretation of mammograms and in their recommendations for management[1]. The reported sensitivity and specificity of mammography vary from 55-94% and 88-99% respectively[2]. The current approach to the mammographic lesion that is difficult to interpret, is to secure a wire into the site of the lesion, tether it and ask the surgeon to perform an excision biopsy. Whereas the former attitude of the surgeon was to excise all lumps in the breast on the grounds that some are malignant, the current approach is to reduce the number of operations for non-malignant breast lesions to as few as possible. To this end, making the distinction between benign and malignant lesions is even more important.

Metastatic spread from breast cancer can involve a variety of organs. One of the common sites is bone and bone scintigraphy plays a major part in evaluating these lesions. This role of nuclear medicine has been discussed in previous series[2] and will not be addressed in this section.

99mTc-MIBI

A new approach to the 'difficult' mammogram is the use of 99mTc-MIBI imaging for the detection of primary breast cancer (Fig 8.1) in association with mammography. Early results of Khalkhali et

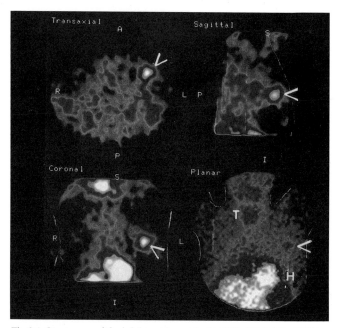

Fig 8.1 *Carcinoma of the left breast imaged with ⁹⁹ᵐTc-MIBI. The SPET images (upper left and right and lower left panels) show focal uptake in the primary tumour (arrowhead). Lower right panel: anterior planar view of the chest showing uptake in the heart H and thyroid T and in the region of the left breast (arrowhead). Courtesy of Dr. Al-Yasi*

al.[3] and Kao et al.[4] showed high sensitivity and specificity for primary breast cancer. More recently, in a large study of 147 women with breast lesions that required biopsies, ⁹⁹ᵐTc-MIBI (740 MBq) was injected and breast images were acquired in the prone and lateral positions. A total of 153 suspicious lesions were evaluated; scintimammography correctly identified cancer in 90% of cases with a 7% false-positive rate and a 3% false-negative rate[5]. Other large multicentre studies evaluating ⁹⁹ᵐTc-MIBI scintimammography are in progress to confirm these early encouraging results. If the findings are replicated then scintimammography may play a complementary role to conventional mammography and reduce the number of biopsies, especially in women with dense breasts and in patients with abnormal lesions on mammography that are not typical of cancer.

However, neither mammography nor ^{99m}Tc-MIBI imaging nor MRI is good for identifying axillary nodal involvement. Since the axillary nodes are no longer excised routinely, a method of identifying their involvement has become important. One approach is to remove only the sentinel node, that is the node nearest the breast cancer. An involved sentinel node on frozen section leads to a further axillary dissection. A normal sentinel node on sampling leads to no further operation, and just a lumpectomy or local excision of the breast tumour is undertaken. The reliability of this approach is questioned and many surgeons feel that a sentinel node is not a reliable indicator of the many lymphatic pathways from the breast to the axilla. Internal mammary nodes tend to be ignored totally on the assumption that it is most unlikely for an internal mammary node to be involved if an axillary node is not involved.

LYMPHOSCINTIGRAPHY

Previous techniques of lymphoscintigraphy using colloids of various sorts for both axillary investigation, either by injection through the finger web or by peri-areola injection, and investigation of the internal mammary nodes by paraxiphisternal injection have not found favour. This is because an involved node is an absence of a normal node. Since such nodes vary considerably, the lack of ability to identify an involved node positively is a major drawback. It is also assumed that a clinically palpable node in the axilla is likely to be involved but the data show that many palpable nodes are merely inflammatory or reactive and do not mean cancer involvement and that many clinically clear axillae have involved nodes in them.

^{18}F-FLUORODEOXYGLUCOSE (^{18}F-FDG) PET IMAGING

Two current imaging techniques have potential for identifying involved axillary (and internal mammary) nodes. One is PET currently using ^{18}F-FDG. With this technique primary breast cancers and malignantly involved nodes are usually positive[6]; however, inflammatory nodes and certain benign tumours also take up this radiopharmaceutical.

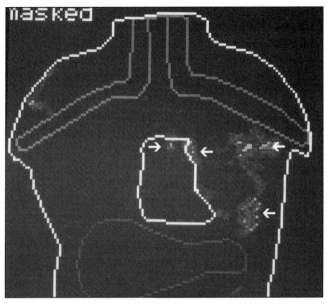

Fig 8.2 *Breast carcinoma with axillary lymph node metastases. Images were acquired with ^{99m}Tc SM3 monoclonal antibody. Probability map in anterior view. 22 h image analysed with respect to changes from 10 min image, with the heart and liver masked out. Left breast and axillary node involvement (areas indicated by ←) is depicted. Courtesy of Dr. M. Granowska*

RADIOIMMUNOSCINTIGRAPHY

The alternative approach is to use a radiolabelled monoclonal antibody capable of binding to surface markers of breast cancer. The results of planar imaging of primary breast cancer and axillary node involvement using radiolabelled monoclonal antibodies [170H.82[7] and anti-CEA[8]] show the latter to be sensitive but insufficiently specific for the purpose.

To improve further the sensitivity of detection and to aid distinction between the involved and the non-involved axillary node, imaging processing has been undertaken using a change detection algorithm. This approach has been successful in more than 90% of cases in a small series in patients with clinically impalpable nodes, half of which were shown correctly to be involved (Fig. 8.2)[9]. It is likely that the combination of specific targeting of a radiolabelled monoclonal antibody and image change detection programmes is likely to be developed further in the future. The use of the peroperative probe in combination with radiolabelled monoclonal antibodies to determine whether there is axillary node involvement at the time of surgery is also being explored.

^{99m}Tc-METHYLENE DIPHOSPHONATE (^{99m}Tc-MDP)

Recently Picollo et al [10] reported the results of ^{99m}Tc-MDP scintimammography. They evaluated 200 patients at high risk for breast cancer. The sensitivity of ^{99m}Tc-MDP scintigraphy was 92%, specificity 95% and accuracy 92% in this selected group of patients. Generally lesions less than 0.7cm were difficult to detect. Tumour to background uptake ratios of the order of 3.8±0.4 were achieved.

A more recent, prospective study compared ^{99m}Tc-MDP and ^{99m}Tc-MIBI scintimammography in patients with equivocal mammographic findings [11]. Sixty-five patients were evaluated. The sensitivity of both imaging modalities was 94%. The specificity of ^{99m}Tc-MIBI was low at 53% while ^{99m}Tc-MDP was 93%.

Imaging of breast cancer and its metastases remains a diagnostic challenge. At present the role of nuclear medicine is limited. Patients with difficult mammograms (microcalcification, the radial scar/complex sclerosing lesion and the presence of atypical ductal or lobular hyperplasia) should be further imaged with ^{99m}Tc-MIBI, ^{99m}Tc-MDP and ^{201}Tl. These scintimammographic techniques help to further differentiate between benign and malignant breast lesions and reduce the number of benign biopsies.

RECEPTOR IMAGING

The radiolabelled receptor binding agents that are used include ^{123}I and ^{18}F oestradiol derivatives for imaging oestrogen receptors and thereby predicting prognosis. The application of radiolabelled monoclonal antibody against the C-ERB2 receptor, the presence of which indicates a poor prognosis, and the use of ^{111}In-pentetreotide (Table 5.1), which is taken up in some breast cancers, are being explored.

The main problem with all the above approaches is that at such a stressful time for the patient, obtaining consent for a new technique involving radioactivity is not easy. The nuclear medicine approach has to be combined and integrated with the total approach to the management of breast cancer by the surgeon.

References

1. Elmore JG, Wells CK, Lee CH et al. Variability in radiologists' interpretations of mammograms. *New England J. of Medicine* 1994; **331**: 1493-1499.

2. McKillop JH, Fogelman I. Oncology. In, Benign and malignant bone disease. Churchill Livingstone, London 1991; 30-52.

3. Khalkhali I, Mena I, Diggles L. Review of imaging techniques for the diagnosis of breast cancer: a new role of probe scintimammography using technetium-99m sestamibi. *European J. of Nuclear Medicine* 1994; **21**: 357-362.

4. Kao CK, Wang SJ, Liu TJ. The use of technetium-99m methoxyisobutyl isonitrile breast scintigraphy to evaluate palpable breast masses. *European J. of Nuclear Medicine* 1994; **21**: 432-436.

5. Khalkhali I, Torrance CA, Cutrone JA et al. Scintimammography versus mammography: complementary role of Tc-99m Sestamibi breast imaging in the prone position for the diagnosis of breast carcinomas. *Radiology* 1994; **193**(S): 158.

6. Wahl RL, Cody R, Hutchins G et al. Primary and metastatic breast carcinoma: Initial clinical evaluation with PET with the radiolabelled glucose analogue 2-[^{18}F]-fluoro-2-deoxy-d-glucose. *Radiology* 1991; **179**: 765-770

7. McEwan AJB, Akram I, Boniface G et al. Tc-99m MoAb 17OH.82 in the evaluation of locoregional disease in patients with breast cancer. *European J. of Nuclear Medicine* 1994; **21**: S15.

8. Lind P, Smola MG, Lechner P et al. The immunoscintigraphic use of Tc-99m-labelled monoclonal anti-CEA antibodies (BW 431/26) in patients with suspected primary recurrent and metastatic breast cancer. *Int. J. of Cancer* 1991; **47**: 865-869.

9. Granowska M, Carroll M, Nimmon CC et al. Radioimmunoscintigraphy, RIS, of breast cancer, BC, using Tc-99m SM3. *European J. of Nuclear Medicine* 1994; **21**: 748.

10. Piccolo S, Lastoria S, Mainolfi C. et al. Technetium-99m methylene diphosphanate scintimammography to image primary breast cancer. *J. of Nuclear Medicine* 1995; **36**: 718-724.

11. Piccolo S, Lastoria S, Varrella P, et al. Comparative results of Tc-99m MIBI and Tc-99m MDP scintimammography in patients with breast abnormalities. *J. of Nuclear Medicine* 1995; **36**: 51P.

Other Tumours

BRAIN TUMOURS

Currently available imaging techniques for brain scanning have improved the clinician's ability to make an early diagnosis, plan treatment and determine brain tumour response to therapy. CT and MRI remain the main imaging modalities for the primary diagnosis of brain tumours. However, both imaging modalities have difficulty in assessing tumour viability after therapy. It is in this context that nuclear medicine imaging techniques such as PET and SPET provide functional information and play an important role[1].

POSITRON EMISSION TOMOGRAPHY

PET investigations of brain tumours have served as the impetus for oncological applications of PET in other organ systems. For PET imaging the most commonly used radiopharmaceutical is ^{18}F-fluorodeoxyglucose (^{18}F-FDG) [dose 185 MBq (5 mCi)]. PET scans provide information about the degree of malignancy and prognosis at presentation. Visual analysis of the images shows increased accumulation of FDG in high-grade tumours while only 10% of low-grade tumours show uptake[2]. The prognosis worsens as the ^{18}F-FDG uptake increases in the tumour: patients with a hypermetabolic tumour have a median survival of 7 months, whereas with normal accumulation or hypometabolic lesions, median survival is 33 months[3].

Following therapy, PET studies with ^{18}F-FDG provide information about residual tumour (Fig 9.1). In a study of 17 patients, increased ^{18}F-FDG accumulation was observed at the surgical margins in 11 patients who showed clinical and CT evidence of recurrence 2 months after surgery[4]. Unlike CT and MRI, PET studies can also differentiate recurrent high-grade malignancies (which show high metabolic rates) from areas of radiation necrosis (which have low metabolic rates)[5,6].

SINGLE-PHOTON EMISSION TOMOGRAPHY

In centres where PET facilities are not available, ^{201}Tl SPET [dose 111-148 MBq (3-4 mCi)] imaging is the most frequently used technique for the evaluation of brain tumours. The exact mechanism for uptake is unknown, but some factors such as the breakdown of blood-brain barrier, change in blood flow and transmembrane active transport into viable cells are considered important in this process. Focal ^{201}Tl uptake appears to correlate well with metabolically active tumour (Fig 9.1)[7]. This information is extremely helpful in directing the surgeon to areas requiring surgical intervention. Another useful application of ^{201}Tl is intraoperative differentiation of tumour from normal brain tissue by using a portable gamma camera system during surgery. This helps the neurosurgeon in complete removal of the tumour. Extensive preoperative ^{201}Tl SPET studies in patients with gliomas have shown that by using a 'threshold index' the grade of the glioma can be predicted with an accuracy of 89%[8]. Lastly, ^{201}Tl SPET imaging can be used to differentiate recurrence of tumour from radiation necrosis; this is an important indication where other diagnostic modalities have limitations[9].

[111]In-pentetreotide has also been used for imaging meningiomas, some gliomas and metastases. The sensitivity of detection for the former tumour is fairly high with this imaging modality. More recently ^{99m}Tc-MIBI has also been used to differentiate between tumour relapse and tumour necrosis and showed a sensitivity of 81%[10]. Further, well-designed studies are required to determine the appropriate role for these techniques in proper management of patients with brain tumours.

HEAD AND NECK TUMOURS

Cancers of head and neck are increasing in frequency and are commonly associated with the use/abuse of alcohol and tobacco. The defined regions include the nasal cavity, paranasal sinuses,

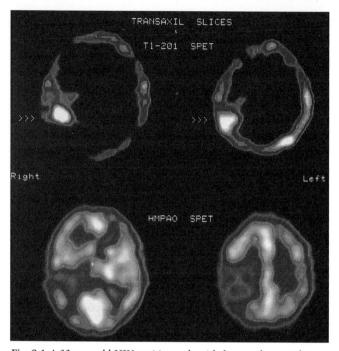

Fig. 9.1 *A 32-year-old HIV-positive male with fever and a mass lesion seen in the right parietal lobe on brain MRI. Anti-Toxoplasma therapy failed to reduce the volume of this lesion. MRI could not establish the differential diagnosis between toxoplasmosis and lymphoma. A ^{201}Tl SPET study was performed (upper panels show transaxial slices). Focal increased tracer uptake is noted (arrowheads) in the right posterior temporoparietal region (tumour/background ratio = 3.0), compatible with lymphoma. Corresponding ^{99m}Tc-HMPAO images show a large perfusion deficit in the same location. (Courtesy of Dr. Durval C. Costa)*

nasopharynx, oral cavity and the oropharynx. The predominant lesion within these defined regions is squamous cell carcinoma.

The clinical requirements are to detect locoregional spread of nasopharyngeal and buccal cancers and identify lymph node involvement. Because of the frequency of tonsillitis and other mouth infections, head and neck lymph nodes are often enlarged. Thus x-ray CT does not in any way confirm the presence of malignancy in these nodes. Furthermore, it is not

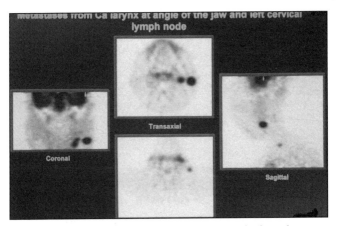

Fig. 9.2 *Carcinoma of the larynx. ^{18}F-FDG PET study showed hypermetabolic focii localised to the left jaw angle and left cervical lymph node*

always possible radiologically to differentiate between tumour and oedematous and/or scarred tissue. Registration of CT/MR and PET images may alter management in these patients and provide the information which can result in more precise planning of surgery. ^{18}F-FDG PET imaging has the potential to detect tumour viability (Fig 9.2)[11]. However, during the period of inflammation secondary to radiation therapy, ^{18}F-FDG accumulation may become diffuse at the therapeutic site and tumour metabolism may be difficult to evaluate. Furthermore, infected glands also take up ^{18}F-FDG.

Radiolabelled MoAbs reacting with squamous cell cancers have been used for imaging. Recently ^{99m}Tc-labelled MoAb E48 IgG and its F(ab')^2 fragment have been used and an accuracy of 81% for lesion detection has been reported[12]. MoAb 174H.64 (from Biomira, Tru-scint SQ) has also detected these tumours and a sensitivity of 88% has been reported[13].

Other radiopharmaceuticals such as ^{99m}Tc-DMSA(V) have also been used to localise these lesions, but the accuracy for detection was poor.

MELANOMAS

Cutaneous melanomas

Cutaneous melanoma is becoming a common disease. In the majority of cases diagnosis of the primary lesion is straightforward. However, evaluation of metastatic disease remains a problem. Extensive radiographic screening rarely reveals metastases in the absence of symptoms and signs, or abnormal liver function test. In this context a test which can identify occult metastases would be very useful. Nuclear medicine provides some techniques which address this problem. Initially ^{67}Ga was used for detecting these lesions; however, the sensitivity and specificity of this test were low. The most encouraging results have been obtained with radiolabelled monoclonal antibodies. In a large multicentre trial involving 254 patients and using ^{99m}Tc-MoAb 225.28S for imaging, it was shown that 70% of the lesions could be identified. Of particular interest was the detection of occult disease in 60 patients[14]. More recently, ^{123}I-$^{(S)}$-2-hydroxy-3-iodo-6-methoxy-^{N}[(1-ethyl-2-pyrrolidinyl)methyl] benzamide (IBZM) has also been employed (Fig. 9.3)[15]. Early results have been encouraging, and further large prospective studies will define the role of this new radiopharmaceutical.

^{18}F-FDG PET scintigraphy has also been used to locate these tumours and their metastases[16]. Scintigraphy correctly identified 15/15 intra-abdominal and lymph node metastases. PET was not as sensitive as CT for small lesions in the lungs. However, of particular interest were the small bowel metastases identified by PET scintigraphy. These bowel lesions are extremely difficult to identify by any method other than surgery or autopsy.

UVEAL MELANOMAS

In occular oncology malignant melanoma is the most frequently encountered tumour. Clinical manifestations of this neoplasm are usually absent unless the macula is involved or retinal detachment has occurred. The ophthalmoscopic diagnosis of uveal melanomas may be reinforced by

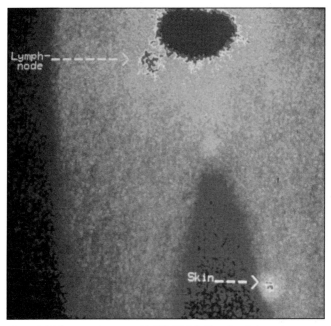

Fig. 9.3 *Melanoma: images with* [123]*I-IBZM. Two focal sites of increased uptake are seen, one to the right of the bladder and another in the inner left thigh. (Courtesy of Dr. Maffioli, National Cancer Institute, Milan and the European Journal of Nuclear Medicine)*

documenting growth on serial photography, by fluorescein fundus angiography and by ultrasonography. In 95% of these lesions diagnosis is not a problem. However, misdiagnosis can occur and opaque media can make direct visualisation virtually impossible. Commonly the tumour may be non-pigmented and it may be difficult to differentiate between a small amelanotic melanoma, a choroidal haemangioma, a choroidal osteoma and a metastasis from an occult primary. It is in this context that nuclear medicine provides imaging techniques to investigate these tumours non-invasively. Phosphorus-32 (^{32}P) has been the most widely used technique for imaging these tumours; however, the technique is cumbersome, which has limited its use in clinical practice. ^{99m}Tc-labelled MoAb 225.28S has been the most widely used MoAb for this purpose (Fig 9.4). With appropriate

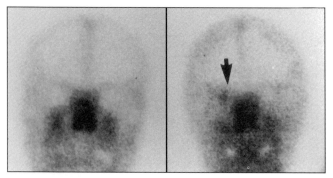

Fig. 9.4 *Anterior skull projection. Images with* ^{99m}*Tc-labelled monoclonal antibody 225.28S (Fab')2 fragments. The image in the left panel shows a normal scan acquired 5 h postinjection. The image in the right panel shows a focal area of increased tracer uptake in the right occular region corresponding to an amelanotic occular melanoma*

technique the reported sensitivity of this method ranges between 86% and 93% and specificity between 93% and 95%[17].

LIVER

Conventional liver scintigraphy performed with ^{99m}Tc-colloid, planar and SPET images has been largely superseded by CT, ultrasonography and MRI. However, in a few clinical conditions scintigraphy provides useful information.

Focal fatty deposits and focal nodular hyperplasia are examples where a hepatic mass detected on CT scan can occasionally be mistaken for a malignant lesion. It should be noted that focal fat deposits in the liver do not produce a mass effect, while focal nodular hyperplasia does. In these cases a liver scan should be performed after an intravenous injection of ^{99m}Tc-colloid [dose 80 MBq (2.1 mCi)]. A combination of a normal ^{99m}Tc-colloid scan and a mass lesion on CT suggests a diagnosis of focal nodular hyperplasia, whereas a normal scintigram with an infiltrating (non-mass-like) appearance of low density on CT suggests focal fatty liver[18,19]. A second type of hepatic lesion that may have a non-specific CT appearance is cavernous haemangioma. In these cases a more definitive diagnosis needs to be obtained since a biopsy can lead to massive haemorrhage. This can be achieved by ^{99m}Tc-labelled RBC radionuclide study of the liver. Birnbaum and Weinreb[20] compared MRI with radiolabelled RBCs in 37 patients who had 69 suspected haemangiomas initially detected by CT or ultrasonography. They found that MRI had a 20% false-positive rate, while radionuclide study was categorically capable of distinguishing haemangiomas from hypervascular metastases. They concluded that ^{99m}Tc-labelled RBC radionuclide study is the method of choice for diagnosing haemangiomas and that MRI should be reserved for diagnosing tiny lesions (less than 2 cm), where the radionuclide study was found to have limitations.

Hepatocellular carcinoma (HCC) is a highly malignant tumour and patients with this tumour have a poor prognosis. Interventional therapy, such as transcatheter arterial chemoembolisation, is considered to be an effective palliative treatment in patients with inoperable HCC. However, after embolisation it is difficult to assess tumour viability. To this end ^{18}F-FDG PET scintigraphy has been used and appears to be a valuable method to assess tumour viability[21].

In the case of hepatic metastases, especially colorectal hepatic metastases, chemotherapy with 5-fluorouracil has been extensively used. However, response rates have varied from 8-82%. Based on a literature survey, Kemeny reported that the average response rate for hepatic metastases was 23%[22]. It is in this context that nuclear medicine techniques can provide extremely useful information in selecting patients who would show a good response to therapy. This is achieved by labelling fluorouracil with [18]F. It was shown that patients with concentration values (SUV) of ^{18}F-FU exceeding 3.5 showed tumour regression while those with lower values did not show any response[23].

HIV-RELATED NEOPLASMS

Kaposi's sarcoma and lymphoma are the main tumours occurring in HIV disease. [201]Tl and ^{67}Ga scintigraphy are the two methods which have evolved to assess these tumours. In our experience, ^{201}Tl whole-body scan provides a good screening procedure for Kaposi's sarcoma, where the neoplasms show increased tracer uptake; subsequently tailored CT or MRI is performed to obtain morphological information. However, to differentiate between pulmonary Kaposi's sarcoma and thoracic lymphoma and infection, sequential ^{201}Tl/^{67}Ga scintigraphy can be performed on the basis that ^{201}Tl localises Kaposi's sarcoma and lymphoma and ^{67}Ga localises in lymphoma and infection only.

SARCOMAS

Soft tissue and bone sarcomas generally carry a poor prognosis. The lung is the most frequent site for metastases followed by bone and liver. For most sarcomas, complete surgical resection is recommended if it can be achieved without excessive morbidity. However, despite adequate treatment a large number of patients with high-grade sarcomas develop metastases. [67]Ga scans have been used both for initial staging and monitoring response to therapy [24]. [67]Ga scintigraphy has a high sensitivity (85%) for detecting these lesions, and the intensity of uptake generally corresponds to the grade of tumour. The more important clinical indication is to assess response of tumour to preoperative chemotherapy. To this end ^{201}Tl and ^{99m}Tc-MIBI have been used [25,26,27]. Both radiopharmaceuticals are good indicators of tumour viability and serial scans show good correlation between uptake and the degree of tumour necrosis on histology.

References

1. Riccabona G. Brain tumour scanning revisited. *Nuclear Medicine Comms.* 1994; **15**: 125-127.

2. DiChiro G. Positron emission tomography using [^{18}F]fluorodeoxyglucose in brain tumours: a powerful diagnostic and prognostic tool. *Investigational Radiology* 1986; **22**: 360-371.

3. Alavi JB, Alavi A, Chawluk J et al. Positron emission tomography in patients with glioma: a predictor of prognosis. *Cancer* 1988; **62**: 1074-1078.

4. Hanson MW, Hoffman JM, Glantz MJ et al. FDG PET in the early postoperative evaluation of patients with brain tumour. *J. of Nuclear Medicine* 1990; **31**: 799.

5. Doyle WK, Budinger TF, Valk PE, Levin VA, Gutin PH. Differentiation of cerebral radiation necrosis from tumour recurrence by ^{18}F-FDG and [82]Rb positron emission tomography. *J. of Computer Assisted Tomography* 1987; **11**: 563-570.

6. DiChiro G, Oldfield E, Wright DC et al. Cerebral necrosis after radiotherapy and/or intrarterial chemotherapy for brain tumours, PET and neuropathologic studies. *Am. J. of Radiology* 1988; **150**: 189-197.

7. Kaplan WD, Takronan T, Morris A et al, Thallium-201 brain tumour imaging: A comparative study with pathologic correlation. *J. of Nuclear Medicine* 1987; **28**: 47-52.

8. Black KL, Hawkins RA, Kim TK et al. Use of thallium-201 SPECT to quantitate malignancy grade of gliomas. *J. of Neurosurgery* 1989; **71**: 342-346.

9. Biersack HJ, Grunwald F, Kropp J. Single photon emission computed tomography imaging of brain tumours. *Seminars in Nuclear Medicine* 1991; **21**: 2-10.

10. Maffioli L, Gasparini M, Castellani MR et al. Tc-99m SestaMIBI SPET in detecting brain tumour relapses. *European J. of Nuclear Medicine* 1994; **21**: 789.

11. Strauss LG, Conti PS. The application of PET in clinical oncology. *J. of Nuclear Medicine* 1991; **32**: 623-648.

12. deBree R, Roos JC, Quak JJ et al. Clinical imaging of head and neck cancer with technetium-99m-labelled monoclonal antibody E48 IgG or F(ab')[2]. *J. of Nuclear Medicine* 1994; **35**: 775-783.

13. Akram I, Jha N, MacLean G et al. Radioimmunoscintigraphy with MAb-174H.64 in patients with head and neck cancers. *European J. of Nuclear medicine* 1994; **21**: S15.

14. Siccardi AG, Buraggi GL, Callegaro L et al. Multicentre study of immunoscintigraphy with radiolabelled monoclonal antibody in patients with melanoma. *Cancer Research* 1986; **46**: 4817-4822.

15. Maffiolo L, Mascheroni L, Mongioj V et al. Scintigraphic detection of melanoma metastases with radiolabelled benzamide ([iodine-123]-(S)-IBZM). *J. of Nuclear Medicine* 1994; **35**: 1741-1747.

16. Gritters LS, Francis IR, Zasadny KR, Wahl RL. Initial assessment of positron emission tomography using 2–fluorine-18-fluoro-2-deoxy-d-glucose in the imaging of malignant melanoma. *J. of Nuclear Medicine* 1993; **34:** 1420-1427.

17. Bomanji J, Hungerford JL, Britton KE. Radioimmunoscintigraphy of ocular melanomas. In Human Melanoma (ed: S. Ferrone) *Springer-Verlag,* London 1990; 373-386.

18. Welch TJ, Sheedy PF, Johnson CM et al. Focal nodular hyperplasia and hepatic adenoma: comparison of angiography, CT, US and scintigraphy. *Radiology* 1985; **156:** 593-595.

19. Halvorsen RA, Thompson WM. Imaging primary and metastatic cancer of the liver. *Seminars in Oncology* 1991; **18:** 111-122.

20. Birnbaum BA, Weinreb JC. Hepatic haemangioma: a comparison of Tc-99m labelled-RBC SPECT and MRI for definitive diagnosis. *Radiology* 1990; **176:** 95.

21. Torizuka T, Tamaki N, Inokuma T et al. Value of fluorine-18-FDG-PET to monitor hepatocellular carcinoma after interventional therapy. *J. of Nuclear Medicine* 1994; **35:** 1965-1969.

22. Kemeny N. The systemic chemotherapy of hepatic metastases. *Seminars of Oncology* 1983; **10:** 148-149.

23. Strauss LG, Conti PS. The application of PET in clinical oncology. *J. of Nuclear Medicine* 1991 **32:** 623-648.

24. Southee AE, Kaplan WD, Jochelson MS, et al. Gallium-67 imaging in metastatic and recurrent soft-tissue sarcoma. *J. of Nuclear Medicine* 1990; **32:** 1594-1599.

25. Ramannah L, Waxman AD, Binney G, et al. Thallium-201 scintigraphy in bone sarcoma: comparison of gallium-67 and technetium-99m MDP in the evaluation of chemotherapy response. *J. of Nuclear Medicine* 1990; **31:** 567-572.

26. Nagaraj N, Ashok G, Waxman A, et al. Clinical usefulness of serial Tc-99m sestamibi (MIBI) scintigraphy in evaluating tumour response to preop chemotherapy in patients with bone and soft tissue sarcomas. *J. of Nuclear Medicine* 1995; **35**: 129P

27. Lin J, Leung W-t, Ho SKW, et al. Quantitative evaluation of thallium-201 uptake in predicting chemotherapeutic response of osteosarcoma. *European J. of Nuclear Medicine* 1995; **22**: 553-555

Basic Principles of Radionuclide Therapy

INTRODUCTION

Radionuclides have been used in therapy for as long as they have been in use for diagnostic purposes. Radionuclide therapy works by the principle of internal targeting.

This approach theoretically permits large radiation doses to be delivered to the tumour target with sparing of the surrounding normal tissue.

For an effective radiation dose to be delivered to the target tissue, high tumour uptake is required, and for a high therapeutic ratio a high tumour to background ratio of the radiopharmaceutical must be achieved. The efficacy of the radiopharmaceutical is also dependent on the tumour residence time. A further factor affecting the dose delivered to the tumour is the nature of the radiation, that is whether the radionuclide delivers beta or alpha radiation, and decays by internal conversion or with the release of Auger electrons.

The principles underlying the choice of radiopharmaceuticals for therapy, the mechanisms of uptake of these agents into tumour sites and their clinical role will be discussed in the following chapters. Some of the radiopharmaceuticals have already been mentioned as diagnostic agents in the preceding chapters and some duplication will therefore be found, but this duplication serves to enable each chapter to be read without reference to others.

PHYSICAL PROPERTIES OF THERAPEUTIC RADIONUCLIDES

Unlike radionuclides used for diagnostic imaging, which are gamma emitters, therapeutic radionuclides emit radiation with a high linear energy transfer (LET), which is able to destroy tumour tissue. Radionuclides that also emit a small quantity of gamma rays (less than 10%) have the advantage that they can be imaged to ensure good tumour uptake prior to embarking on therapy. Gamma emissions in high abundance, however, are undesirable as they contribute to the whole-body radiation burden of the patient and are a source of unwanted radiation to staff and family members.

Radionuclides that may be used for therapy fall into three main categories:

1) Beta-emitting radionuclides
2) Alpha-emitting radionuclides
3) Electron capture and internal conversion decaying radionuclides

Beta-Emitting Radionuclides

Beta-emitting radionuclides are at present the only type of radionuclide to be used clinically. Beta particles deposit their radiation dose within a few millimetres and thereby spare surrounding normal tissue. The range of beta particles is from 200 μm to several mm.

Alpha-Emitting Radionuclides

Alpha particles deliver a high radiation dose over a short distance (80 keV per μm) and have an extremely short range when compared with beta particles (50-90 μm). The alpha-emitting radionuclides that could be used clinically are few as most have complex decay schemes. Astatine-211 is the most promising.

Electron Capture and Internal Conversion Decaying Radionuclides

In both electron capture and internal conversion an inner shell electron vacancy is created within the atom which is filled from an outer shell with release of Auger electrons or low-energy x-rays. The range of these low-energy particles is extremely short (less than 1 μm). This approach requires internalisation of

	T 1/2	Emax (MeV)	Gamma energies (keV)
Iodine-131	8.1 days	0.6	637, 364
Yttrium-90	2.7 days	2.3	-
Phosphorus-32	14.3 days	1.7	-
Samarium-153	46.3 h	0.8	103
Strontium-89	50.5 days	1.5	-
Rhenium-186	3.7 days	1.07	137

Table 10.1 *Physical properties of therapeutic radionuclides used in clinical practice*

the radionuclide for efficacy in biological systems.

The physical half-life of a radionuclide to be used for therapy should fit with the biological half-life of the radiopharmaceutical in the tumour. However, a long physical half-life is appropriate if the radionuclide is released on or into the tumour by its carrier. A list of therapeutic radionuclides currently in use, together with their physical characteristics, is shown in Table 10.1.

RADIOBIOLOGY

Whilst much is understood about the radiobiological effects of external beam radiation which is delivered in a fractionated protocol, little work has been undertaken to determine the radiobiological effects of continuous low-dose, low-dose-rate radiation administered internally.

Unlike external beam radiotherapy where the dose is delivered to a defined area, the distribution of the targeted radiotherapy dose will depend on the blood supply to and within the tumour and also on the homogeneity of the tumour mass. Targeted radiotherapy is also dependent on the viability of the tumour cell, particularly if the radiopharmaceutical is to be internalized within the tumour cell.

Low LET and low-dose radiation may cause initial damage

which is subsequently modified by post-irradiation cellular processes such as repair. The ability of tumour tissue to repair after radionuclide therapy has been poorly studied.

Radiosensitivity is another significant factor affecting the response of tumour cells to radionuclide therapy.
Hypoxic cells are recognised as being relatively radioresistant. As yet, little work has been undertaken to attempt to improve the efficacy of radionuclide therapy by using a radiosensitiser in conjunction with a therapeutic radiopharmaceutical. Studies in which the cell cycling rate is altered to improve radiosensitivity have also not as yet been undertaken.

DOSIMETRY

The MIRD schema is the accepted method for calculating a tumour radiation dose from internally administered radiopharmaceuticals. It is also used to calculate the radiation dose received by normal tissues[1].

The method of calculating the radiation dose to the tumour assumes two sources of radiation. The first is the source of radiation that is within the tumour target and the second is the radiation from the surrounding normal tissue.

The main sources of error in dosimetric calculations are that they assume a uniform distribution of the radiopharmaceutical within the target, which is rare given the heterogeneous nature of tumours and their blood supply. The second source of error is the assumptions that must be made about tumour volumes. The MIRD schema also do not distinguish between a radiopharmaceutical that is bound to the tumour cell membrane, one that is internalised within the tumour cell and one that is localised within the tissue adjacent to the tumour. Since the tumour cell nucleus is the target 'organ' a calculation of dose to the nucleus would be more relevant than a calculation of dose to the tumour as a whole. The mean dose to the tumour cell nucleus will obviously vary depending on whether the therapeutic radiopharmaceutical is internalised within the cell close to the nucleus or localised outside the tumour cell.

MECHANISMS OF RADIOPHARMACEUTICAL LOCALISATION

Radiopharmaceuticals localise via a variety of mechanisms either within the tumour cells or within the surrounding normal tissues.

Internal localisation of therapeutic radiopharmaceuticals within a tumour cell can only occur if the agent is able to cross the membrane of the cell and is then bound within the cytoplasm or to the nuclear DNA.

An excellent example of a therapeutic radiopharmaceutical which is internalised within the tumour cell is iodine-131 (^{131}I). ^{131}I is taken up by differentiated follicular thyroid cancer cells in which it is metabolised. The beta radiation dose is delivered not only within the tumour cell, leading to cell death, but also to neighbouring cells. The degree of uptake depends on the extent to which the tumour cell continues to exhibit the metabolic features of the normal thyroid follicular cell.

^{131}I-metaiodobenzylguanidine (^{131}I-MIBG) is another radiopharmaceutical that is taken up into tumour cells. MIBG is a guanethidine analogue that is taken up into the neurosecretory granules found in many neuroendocrine cancer cells such as phaeochromocytoma.

As well as incorporation into the metabolic pathways of tumour cells, radiopharmaceuticals may be internalised by utilising the DNA binding properties of certain chemicals. The DNA binding utility of bleomycin has been used in the development of therapeutic agents. The results have been disappointing, however, as the tumour to non-tumour ratio of the labelled compound is significantly less than that of the unlabelled compound[2].

Binding to the cell membrane is another mechanism for localising radiopharmaceuticals. Radiolabelled monoclonal antibodies to a wide variety of antigens localised on the tumour cell membrane have been developed. At present most of the antibodies are not entirely tumour specific and react with antigens found on some normal tissues. This reduces the radiation dose to the tumour target and increases the unwanted effects on normal tissues.

Another mechanism for localising radiopharmaceuticals to tumour cell membranes is to take advantage of the receptors that are present on some tumour cells. Somatostatin receptors are found on a large number of tumour cells including neuroendocrine tumours (see Gastroendocrine tumours section). Although at present only diagnostic radiopharmaceuticals have been designed to image tumours bearing these receptors, the potential exists for the development of therapeutic agents binding to somatostatin receptors.

Localisation of a radiopharmaceutical within or adjacent to tumour tissue is a further mechanism even though no specific uptake or binding of the radiopharmaceutical has occurred. The radiopharmaceutical may be introduced into the capillary bed of the tumour in the form of radiolabelled microspheres. Microspheres are 10 μm in diameter and embolise the tumour when they are delivered into the capillary bed. The degree of degradability of the microspheres and the rate of degradation must be modified taking into account the half-life of the therapeutic radionuclide. Yttrium-90 glass microspheres are an example of such a therapeutic radiopharmaceutical.

Therapeutic doses of radionuclide may be localised close to the tumour by utilising uptake mechanisms in adjacent non–tumour tissue. A number of different radiopharmaceuticals have been developed for the palliative treatment of bone metastases. These agents are taken up into the osteoblasts in the reactive bone adjacent to the tumour sites. These agents include ^{32}P, ^{89}Sr, samarium-153 ethylene diamine tetramethylene diphosphate (^{153}Sm EDTMP) and rhenium-186 hydroxyethylidene diphosphonate (^{186}Re HEDP).

Finally, localisation of therapeutic radiopharmaceuticals may be achieved using intracavitary administration of agents. Yttrium-90, gold-198 and phosphorus-32 have been used for intracavity therapy in colloidal forms. The use of beta particles emitted from the radionuclide in contact with the affected tissue surface gives a high radiation dose with the resultant palliation of malignant effusions. Radiolabelled antibodies have also been used to treat ascites from ovarian cancer following intraperitoneal administration.

Location	Example
Intracellular	^{131}I
	^{131}I-MIBG
	^{131}I- Lipiodol
	^{32}P-phosphorus
Membrane Bound	^{131}I-monoclonal antibodies
Extracellular	^{90}Y microspheres
	^{89}Sr
	^{153}Sm-EDTMP
	^{186}Re-HEDP

Table 10.2 *Mechanisms of localisation of therapeutic radiopharmaceuticals*

A summary of the mechanisms of localisation of therapeutic radiopharmaceuticals is provided in Table 10.2.

References

1. MIRD Medical International Radiation Dose Committee Society of Nuclear Medicine.

2. Beer H, Blauenstein P, Andres R, Hasler P, Schubiger P. How to get the radionuclide to the right site. In: Schubiger P and Hasler PH (eds) Radionuclides for therapy. Proc of the 4th Bottenstein Colloquium, Basle, Hoffman la Roche 1986; 60-74.

Iodine-131 Therapy for Carcinoma of the Thyroid

INTRODUCTION

Iodine-131 (^{131}I) has been used in the treatment of benign thyroid disease for more than forty years. In the past 20 years its use in the treatment of patients with differentiated thyroid cancer has become established. It is the success of ^{131}I in this disease that has stimulated the development of other radiopharmaceuticals for the treatment of malignancy.

IODINE-131

^{131}I is produced by the fission of uranium-235 and by the neutron bombardment of stable tellurium in a nuclear reactor. It decays by the emission of gamma radiations (see Table 10.1) and has a half-life of 8.1 days.

The main advantages of ^{131}I in the form of sodium iodide are its cheapness and its relative availability whilst its main disadvantage is the high-energy gamma emissions which have radiation protection implications for staff, patients and relatives.

^{131}I is administered orally, either as liquid or in the form of a capsule. In rare cases an intravenous preparation may be used.

CLINICAL ROLE OF ^{131}I IN THYROID CANCER

^{131}I has two main therapeutic roles in thyroid cancer. The first is the ablation of residual normal thyroid tissue following surgery, and the second is the treatment of recurrent disease.

Thyroid ablation

Following surgery for a thyroid nodule and histological confirmation of malignancy, ablation of residual thyroid tissue is now an accepted part of management. Ablation both destroys a potential site of malignant recurrence and,

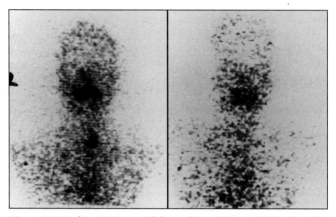

Figure 11.1 *Iodine-131 scans of the neck in a 43 year old female with a papillary carcinoma of the thyroid following surgery to the primary tumour. **Left panel:** shows uptake in the lower left neck in remnant thyroid tissue. **Right panel:** scans performed one year later following successful ablation of the thyroid remnant*

more importantly, facilitates interpretation of uptake in the neck on a diagnostic ^{131}I scan. Ablation of residual thyroid tissue also ensures that subsequent therapeutic doses of ^{131}I will be taken up into recurrent tumour sites.

Although ^{131}I therapy is most useful in patients with follicular thyroid cancer and papillary tumours with follicular elements, ablation of residual thyroid tissue is also undertaken in patients with pure papillary tumours and patients with medullary thyroid cancer.

The dose used for thyroid ablation ranges from 1110 MBq (30 mCi) to 7400 MBq (200 mCi). The lower the dose that is selected, the greater is the probability that additional doses will be required to achieve ablation. The higher doses are accompanied by an increasing incidence of side-effects, particularly when there is a significant amount of residual thyroid tissue. Some centres use a fixed dose for ablation while others adjust the dose according to the size of the remnant demonstrated on a tracer study[1].

Patients requiring ablation should only be treated when levels of thyroid-stimulating hormone (TSH) are high

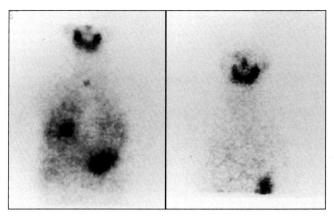

Figure 11.2 *Iodine-131 scans of the neck and anterior thorax in a 75 year old female whose thyroglobulin levels had risen 10 years after thyroidectomy for a follicular thyroid carcinoma.* **Left panel:** *the scan shows uptake of* ^{131}I *in both lung fields more marked on the right.* **Right panel:** ^{131}I *scan performed one year later after two therapy doses of* ^{131}I *showing resolution of lung metastases*

(preferably greater than 30 mIU/l) to ensure optimum uptake of ^{131}I into the gland. This will generally necessitate stopping thyroxine therapy for 1 month before treatment is undertaken (Fig 11.1)

Treatment of recurrence

Once the thyroid remnant has been destroyed, uptake seen on a ^{131}I tracer scan that is not due to the normal biodistribution of ^{131}I in the urinary tract, liver, gut and salivary glands can be attributed to tumour recurrence. This can be treated with therapeutic doses of ^{131}I which generally range from 3700 to 5550 MBq (100-150 mCi). Using ^{131}I, extremely high radiation doses to tumour sites may be achieved (Fig. 11.2). The success of therapy has been well documented and both local recurrences and distant metastases, including those to the lung, respond to therapy[1]. Bone metastases, however, appear more resistant to treatment[2].

Doses up to 16.6 GBq (450 mCi) have been administered with no reported permanent damage to the bone marrow. Patients with widespread metastases should be treated with caution as suppression of leucocytes and platelets may occur. The suppression is transient, however, and rarely requires transfusion.

In patients with large volumes of recurrent tumour, surgical debulking should be performed, if possible prior to ^{131}I administration. Repeat treatments should be given at intervals of usually not less than 6 months to patients whose tracer scan continues to be positive for recurrent disease.

As with thyroid ablation, thyroxine therapy should be discontinued for 1 month (and therapy with triiodothyronine for 2 weeks) before treatment to allow TSH levels to rise. Some groups also recommend the use of a low-iodine diet in the month preceeding treatment to enhance ^{131}I uptake by the tumour cells. Thyroxine therapy may be recommenced 1 week after treatment.

Side-effects of treatment

Side-effects from ^{131}I therapy are remarkably low. The most common of the early side-effects is discomfort in the salivary glands. This radiation sialitis is generally short-lived although some patients may complain of a permanent alteration in taste. Some patients may complain of nausea 24-48 h after administration. This symptom is rarely severe and responds well to simple anti-emetics.

Although oligospermia and azoospermia have been reported[3], long-term studies show no increased incidence of infertility[4]. Leukaemia has been reported as a late side-effect in a limited number of patients, all of whom received high doses at intervals of less than 6 months[5].

Radiation protection issues

As ^{131}I is a high-energy gamma emitter, patients treated with therapeutic doses of ^{131}I constitute a radiation hazard. The regulations vary throughout Europe but in most countries admission and isolation are a legal requirement. The period of admission in a purpose-designed room with a self-contained toilet and shower is generally only 3 days. Drinking large volumes of liquid and encouraging regular bladder emptying aids clearance of excreted ^{131}I and reduces the radiation dose to the bladder. Regular showering reduces skin contamination from ^{131}I excreted in sweat. Disposable sheets, cups and plates should be used. These and other waste should be collected, monitored and stored until below the permitted level for disposal. Visitors and nursing attendance are restricted according to local systems of work. Daily monitoring of the radiation levels should be undertaken until levels fall below the nationally defined limits for discharge and for transport home. Precautions, as set out in an instruction booklet given to the patient, should be explained and continued for a week after discharge; the precautions include absence from work and the avoidance of pregnant women and small children. Pregnancy should be avoided for 6 months after treatment.

References

1. O'Doherty MJ, Nunan TO, Croft DN. Radionuclides and therapy of thyroid cancer. *Nuclear Medicine Comms* 1993; **14:** 736-755.

2. Brown AP, Greening WP, McCready VR, Shaw HJ, Harmer CL. Radioiodine treatment of metastatic thyroid carcinoma: the Royal Marsden Hospital experience. *Brit. J. of Radiology* 1984; **57:** 323-327.

3. Dobyns BM, Sheline GE, Workman J, Tompkins AE, McConahey WM, Becker DV. Malignant and benign neoplasms of the thyroid to patients treated for hyperthyroidism. A report of the Cooperative thyrotoxicosis. Follow up study. *J. of Clin. Endocrinology and Metabolism* 1974; **38:** 976-998.

4. Sarker S, Beierwaltes WH, Gill SP, Contey BJ. Subsequent fertility and birth histories of children and adolescents treated with 131-iodine for thyroid cancer. *J. of Nuclear Medicine* 1976; **17:** 460-464.

5. Edmonds C, Smith T. The long term hazards of treatment of thyroid cancer with radioiodine. *Brit. J. of Radiology* 1986; **59:** 45-51.

^{131}I-MIBG in the Treatment of Neuroectodermal Tumours

INTRODUCTION

^{131}I-metaiodobenzylguanidine (^{131}I-MIBG) was developed initially as a diagnostic agent for detecting benign and malignant phaeochromocytomas[1]. Since then the therapeutic uses of this agent have been explored in a wide variety of neuroectodermal tumours. These tumours are characterised by the active uptake 1 mechanism at the cell membrane which transports the tracer into the storage granules in the cytoplasm. Up to 95% of patients with phaeochromocytomas, 92% with neuroblastomas, 71% with carcinoid tumours and 35% with medullary thyroid cancers[2,3,4,5] take up MIBG into their tumours (Table 12.1).

^{131}I-MIBG THERAPY FOR MALIGNANT PHAEOCHROMOCYTOMA

Malignant phaeochromocytoma has a poor prognosis since these tumours are generally resistant to radiotherapy and chemotherapy. Surgery remains the first-line treatment for primary disease, but metastatic recurrences are frequently multiple and inoperable. The prognosis is worse in patients whose tumours secrete catecholamines which cause hypertensive episodes.

Since more than 90% of malignant phaeochromocytomas take up ^{131}I-MIBG (Fig. 12.1), therapy with this radiopharmaceutical has now been undertaken in a large number of patients, with over one-third experiencing a partial response and some, a complete[6]. The most impressive results relate to subjective symptomatic response. This is probably due to the effectiveness of ^{131}I-MIBG therapy in reducing catecholamine secretion.

^{131}I-MIBG uptake	No ^{131}I-MIBG uptake
Phaeochromocytomas	Insulinomas
Neuroblastomas	Gastrinomas
Carcinoids	VIPomas
Medullary thyroid cancers	
Paragangliomas	

Table 12.1 *Neuroendocrine tumours reported either to take up or not to take up* ^{131}I-MIBG

Therapeutic doses administered to patients have ranged from 3.7-11 GBq (100-300 mCi), but the more recently reported results have favoured the use of higher doses. Treatment has been repeated at intervals ranging from 6 weeks to 3 months[7] and since a therapeutic response may not be obtained until the second or third dose, therapy should be continued for up to four doses before being considered to have failed. Partial responses have been maintained for up to 108 months[8,9].

^{131}I-MIBG therapy in neuroblastoma

Neuroblastoma is a relatively common tumour of childhood and the prognosis is extremely variable. Children who are less than 1 year old or who have a TNM stage 1 or 2 tumour with favourable biological features have a 95-100% 3-year survival. Children who are older than 1 year with stage 4 disease or who have unfavourable biological features such as amplified N-myc have a less than 10% chance of long-term survival.

The treatment of neuroblastoma depends on the stage of the disease. Stages 1 and 2 are treated by complete surgical excision while stages 3 and 4 are treated with combination chemotherapy before surgery to the primary lesion. This is followed by further postoperative chemotherapy. External beam radiotherapy may also be used. Although 80% of children will respond to this regimen initially, there is a high level of relapse.

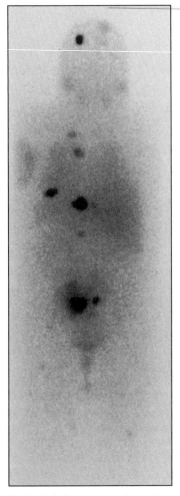

Figure 12.1 ¹²³*I-MIBG whole body image of a patient with malignant phaeochromocytoma. Image shows multiple sites of increased tracer uptake in the skull, lung, spine, para-aortic region and pelvis.*

^{131}I-MIBG has been used to treat children with progressive recurrent disease after failure of conventional therapy. Of the children so treated, 14% experienced a complete remission and a further 48% had a partial response[7]. Early encouraging results have also been reported for ^{131}I-MIBG therapy given just after diagnosis for tumour debulking prior to surgery[8].

^{131}I-MIBG in carcinoid

Carcinoid tumours account for approximately 1% of all malignant gastrointestinal tumours and 10% of these cases are associated with the syndrome of flushing, diarrhoea, and bronchospasm caused by hydroxy indoleacetic acid (5-HIAA) secretion together with other vasoactive peptides. Prognosis of this tumour depends on location and the presence of metastases at the time of presentation. The 5-year survival is 30% or less for patients who have distant metastases[10].

Therapy involves surgery to the primary tumour and isolated liver metastases. Multiple liver metastases are treated by arterial embolization supplemented by interferon or sandostatin therapy. Chemotherapy has been shown to have limited value with high toxicity reported.

^{131}I-MIBG has been used to treat patients in whom all other treatment modalities have failed and with disabling symptoms. Cumulative data showed an incidence of partial response in 20% of patients and palliative responses in more than 50% of patients with end-stage disease[6]. No complete cures have been reported (Fig. 12.2).

^{131}I-MIBG THERAPY IN OTHER NEUROENDOCRINE TUMOURS

Medullary thyroid cancers and paragangliomas are two other neuroendocrine tumours in which ^{131}I-MIBG therapy has been used. Only 30% of the rare medullary thyroid tumours take up ^{131}I-MIBG and opportunities to evaluate its use have therefore been limited. Treatment options are limited to surgery since most of these tumours appear radioresistant. Partial and palliative responses have been reported in the small series in the literature[11] (Fig. 12.3).

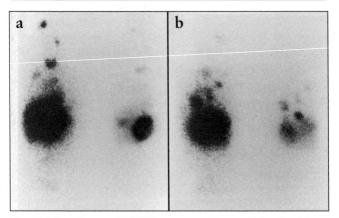

Fig. 12.2 *Post therapy ^{131}I-MIBG scan in a 64 year old female with widespread metastatic carcinoid tumour. (a) anterior high and low intensity scans (b) posterior high and low intensity scans, demonstrating good uptake of therapy dose in known tumour sites including liver, lung, bone and orbital metastases. Following four courses of ^{131}I-MIBG therapy, the liver metastases reduced in size and her syptoms improved*

Experience with paragangliomas is even more limited and case reports only appear in the literature [9, 12]. Again, these are rare tumours and both secreting and non-secreting types exist. Both partial and complete responses have been reported.

Practical aspects of ^{131}I-MIBG therapy

Before administering ^{131}I-MIBG a drug history should be obtained from the patient as a number of drugs significantly interfere with ^{131}I-MIBG uptake. A list of those drugs is given in Table 4.1 and they should be discontinued for at least 2 weeks before therapy.

Thyroid blockade is carried out with oral potassium iodide 60 mg b.d. given 48 h prior to therapy and oral potassium perchlorate 400 mg an hour before infusion to minimize the radiation dose to the thyroid. This is unnecessary in patients with medullary thyroid cancer who have already had a thyroidectomy.

^{131}I-MIBG is administered as a slow intravenous infusion

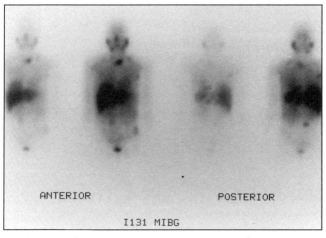

Fig. 12.3 *Post therapy ^{131}I-MIBG scan in a patient with metastatic medullary thyroid cancer. Following this treatment there was a significant fall in calcitonin levels*

over 30-60 min to avoid the theoretical complications of a hypertensive episode in patients with malignant phaeochromocytoma. No such episode has been reported in the literature but ECG, pulse and blood pressure are monitored (using an automatic blood pressure monitor to avoid exposure to staff) throughout the infusion. The doses administered have ranged up to 11 GBq. The recent reports of the results of treatment have suggested that higher doses are more effective in achieving a response. Unfortunately the fact that relatively few patients are suitable for treatment precludes a formal dose escalation trial. The frequency of treatment ranges from monthly for patients with rapidly growing tumours such as neuroblastoma to 6 monthly for patients with slowly growing tumours such as medullary thyroid carcinoma.

The main practical aspects of therapy relate to the radiation protection issues since there are significant potential hazards to staff and other patients unless careful protocols are followed. The use of a designated room with en suite bathroom facilities is mandatory and a dedicated shielded infusion system should be used.

The treatment of children with neuroblastoma requires expertise both in managing a child in an isolated environment and in minimizing radiation doses to parents. The urinary excretion of ¹³¹I-MIBG poses the greatest contamination risk especially in small children. In these patients catheterisation for the duration of hospitalization may be required. Given the potential hazard of ¹³¹I-MIBG therapy it is recommended that therapy is only undertaken in centres that have developed expertise in the area. ¹³¹I-MIBG therapy costs approximately £2500 for a single dose.

SIDE-EFFECTS OF ¹³¹I-MIBG THERAPY

Side-effects of ¹³¹I-MIBG therapy are relatively few and rarely severe. During the infusion of ¹³¹I-MIBG flushing has been observed in some patients with carcinoid syndrome[7]. Nausea may be experienced by some patients during and for 24 h after the infusion due to its iodine content. This is readily relieved by standard anti-emetics and these should be used prophylactically in patients who are being retreated and have had nausea with previous treatment.

Following treatment, falls in platelet and white count have been observed and careful monitoring should be undertaken. The dose-limiting organ for ¹³¹I-MIBG therapy is the bone marrow. This is particularly important in patients who have widespread bone metastases or who have been pretreated with chemotherapy. Generally upon discharge, follow-up should include serial determination of blood count, liver function test, thyroid function test, urinary catecholamines and adrenal glucocorticoid levels.

As with ¹³¹I, women should be told to avoid pregnancy for 6 months after treatment.

References

1. Wieland DM, Brown LE, Mangner TJ, Swanscombe DP, Bierwaltes, W.H. Radiolabelled adrenergic neuron blocking agents: Adrenomedullary imaging with ¹³¹I-iodobenzyl guanidine. *J. of Nuclear Medicine* 1980; **21**: 349-353.

2. Sisson JC, Frager MS, Valk TW et al. Scintigraphic localisation of phaeochromocytoma. *New England J. of Medicine* 1981; **305:** 12-17.

3. Hoefnagel CA. MIBG and somatostatin in oncology: role in the management of neural crest tumours. *European J. of Nuclear Medicine* 1994; **21:** 561-581.

4. Castellani MR, di Bartolomeo M, Maffioli L, Zilembo N, Gasparini M, Buraggi GL. ^{131}I-Iodine MIBG therapy in carcinoid tumours. *J. of Nuclear Medicine and Biology* 1991; **35:** 349-351.

5. Clarke SEM, Lazarus CR, Edwards S, Murby B, Clarke DG, Roden T, Fogelman I, Maisey MN. Scintigraphy and treatment of MTC with ^{131}I-iodine MIBG. *J. of Nuclear Medicine* 1987; **28:** 1820-1824.

6. Shapiro B. Summary, conclusions and future directions of ^{131}I-iodine MIBG therapy in the treatment of neural crest tumours. *J. of Nuclear Medicine and Biology* 1991; **35:** 357-361.

7. Hoefnagel CA, Voute PA, de Kraker J, Valdes Olmos RA. ^{131}I-iodine MIBG therapy after conventional therapy for neuroblastoma. *J. of Nuclear Medicine and Biology* 1991: **35:** 202-207.

8. Hoefnagel CA, de Kraker J, Valdes Olmos RA, Voute PA. ^{131}I-MIBG as a first-line treatment in high-risk neuroblastoma patients. *Nuclear Medicine Comms,* 1994; **15:** 712-717.

9. Bomanji J, Britton KE, Ur E, et al. Treatment of malignant phaeochromocytoma, paraganglioma and carcinoid tumours with metaiodobenzylguanidine. *Nuclear Medicine Comms* 1993; **14:** 856-861.

10. Maton PN. The carcinoid tumour and the carcinoid syndrome. pp1640-1643 in: Becker KL (ed) Principles and Practice of Endocrinology and Metabolism, *Philadelphia, Lippincott* 1990.

11. Clarke SEM. ^{131}I-iodine MIBG in MTC: Guys Hospital Experience. *J. of Nuclear Medicine and Biology* 1991; **35:** 323-327.

12. Baulieu JL, Guilloteau D, Baulieu F. Therapeutic effectiveness of ^{131}I-iodine MIBG on bone metastases of a non-secreting paraganglioma. *J. of Nuclear Medicine* 1988; **29:** 2008–2013.

Radionuclide Therapy of Bone Metastases

INTRODUCTION

Bone metastases are the most common cause of pain in patients with cancer and post-mortem studies show that up to 85% of patients with breast or prostate cancer have bone metastases at the time of death[1]. Patients with bone metastases may survive a number of years in severe pain and with impaired mobility. The causes of bone pain in patients with metastases are complex and the most common are listed in Table 13.1. The amount of pain experienced appears unrelated to the number or size of the metastases.

Palliation of bone pain may be attempted using a number of different modalities. Analgesics in the form of non-steroidal anti-inflammatory drugs and both weak and strong opiates play a major role alone and in conjunction with other therapies. Side-effects of nausea, constipation and drowsiness, however, may require additional medication. Nerve blocks using local anaesthesia or phenol are of use in patients with focal pain. Biphosphonates are also used to palliate pain and are extremely successful in some patients, but symptoms of nausea and vomiting may prove troublesome. The incidence of pathological fractures is reduced in patients treated with biphosphonates and there is a slower development of other complications.

External beam radiotherapy has for many years been one of the mainstays of metastatic bone pain palliation. This may be given as a local dose to a painful area or as a hemibody treatment for patients with bone pain from disseminated lesions. Local radiotherapy is well tolerated and successful in up to 80% of patients treated. Tissue tolerance limits the number of treatments that can be given to any one area. Daily fractionation regimens may necessitate admission of patients for whom daily travel is unacceptable on the grounds of discomfort or distance.

- Stretching of the periosteum overlying the metastases

- Tumour growth into surrounding nerves and soft tissues

- Pathological fracturing

- Prostaglandin release

Table 13.1 *Causes of pain in patients with bone metastases*

Hemibody radiotherapy is a successful treatment for patients with widespread pain. Pain relief is achieved in up to 80% of patients and the onset of relief is usually rapid, within 24-48 h. Side-effects are significant, with nausea, vomiting, diarrhoea, alopecia and radiation pneumonitis following whole body irradiation. Myelosuppression is also a serious side-effect in those patients who require both upper and lower body irradiation.

Many patients with bone metastases have pain at many sites. A systemic treatment therefore has advantages over a local one. An ideal systemic therapy would be a single treatment administered on an outpatient basis which is inexpensive and has no significant side-effects. Radionuclide therapy using strontium-89, samarium-153 EDTMP and rhenium-186 HEDP is able to fulfil some of these criteria.

STRONTIUM-89 (^{89}Sr)

^{89}Sr has been shown to localize in the skeleton at sites of prostatic and breast metastases[2]. The behaviour of intravenous strontium has been studied using ^{85}Sr, which, unlike the pure beta emitter ^{89}Sr, can be imaged as it also emits gamma photons. It has been shown that metastatic bone lesions accumulate and retain strontium more avidly than normal bone.

Although the first reports of the therapeutic use of ^{89}Sr appeared in the early 1940s, it was not until the 1970s that further reports appeared. Since then many studies have been undertaken with this agent in patients with painful metastases from prostate cancer, with reported response rates of 75% and with up to 25% of patients able to discontinue analgesics

101

completely[2,3]. A double-blind trial has been undertaken to assess the placebo effect of ^{89}Sr and has concluded that there is a true therapeutic response to ^{89}Sr that cannot be explained by placebo response[4].

Strontium-89 has been compared with radiotherapy in a controlled multicentre study[5]. Patients were grouped according to their suitability for local or wide-field radiotherapy and were then randomized to receive either ^{89}Sr or radiotherapy. The response was assessed at 3 months and it was shown that ^{89}Sr is as effective as radiotherapy in producing pain relief and may offer the advantage of delaying the onset of pain at new sites. ^{89}Sr is administered as a single intravenous injection. Hospital admission is not necessary. No clear dose-response relationship has been demonstrated but there appears to be a threshold of 1 MBq/kg below which ^{89}Sr is ineffective. There is a response plateau at 1.5-2 MBq/kg above which dose there is increasing toxicity with no further benefit in pain relief. A standard dose of 150 MBq is therefore recommended.

The usual time to onset of pain relief is 10-20 days after injection and the duration of response ranges from 4 to 12 months. Side-effects are minimal. A transient flare pain response has been reported in some patients approximately 48h after injection and this has been regarded as a good prognostic sign. Temporary myelosuppression occurs in some patients, with a nadir at 4-6 weeks and a slow recovery over the next 3-6 weeks. The risk of haematological toxicity is cumulative and haematological monitoring is essential after repeated treatments.

^{89}Sr may safely be used after radiotherapy.

SAMARIUM-153 (^{153}Sm) EDTMP

Samarium-153 EDTMP is a stable compound that concentrates preferentially in skeletal metastases[5]. The relatively short half-life of 46.3 h compared with the long half-life of ^{89}Sr results in a higher dose rate delivery. Furthermore, [153]Sm can also be imaged (Fig. 13.1). Early reports in the literature indicate that [153]Sm-EDTMP can successfully palliate the pain from bone metastases. Turner et al. reported a 79% palliative response in patients with prostatic cancer. Pain palliation occurred within 14 days and lasted up to 35 weeks[6].

Clinical experience with [153]Sm-EDTMP is limited at present to that obtained in phase II and III trials. Doses of 20-40 MBq/kg are currently being used. Treatment is given as a single intravenous injection on an out-patient basis. Symptomatic improvement usually occurs within 2 weeks of treatment with a median duration of benefit of 8 weeks[6]. Repeat treatments have been given at 4-week intervals with response rates of 89%[5].

The advantage of Samarium-153 over Strontium-89 is that bone marrow irradiation is less and Samarium-153 has a short half-life. Thus, therapy can be given more frequently and safely.

RHENIUM-186 ([186]Re) HEDP

Like [153]Sm, [186]Re has a relatively short half-life compared with [89]Sr. Tumour to marrow absorbed doses are double those achieved using [89]Sr[7]. Clinical experience with [186]Re-HEDP is at present extremely limited, but response rates of 80-90% have been reported following a single treatment of 1.2-1.8 GBq in patients with prostate and breast cancer[8]. Like Strontium-89 and Samarium-153, symptom relief is rapid. A pain flare has been observed in 50% of patients treated[9]. Toxicity is limited to temporary myelosuppression with complete recovery by 8 weeks following therapy. A double-blind study of [186]Re-HEDP against ^{99m}Tc-MDP confirmed the therapeutic efficacy of the [186]Re compound[7].

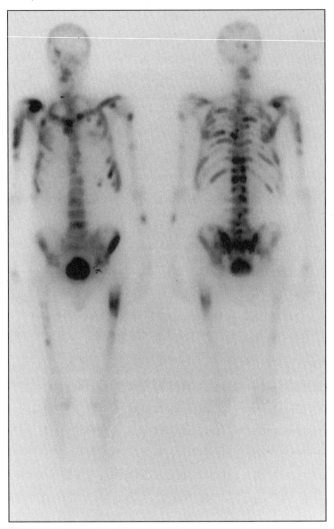

Fig. 13.1 *Patient with carcinoma of the prostate and bone metastases treated with ^{153}Sm-EDTMP (dose 37 MBq/kg). Anterior and posterior whole-body images show multiple focal areas of increased tracer throughout the bony skeleton consistent with widespread bone metastases*

PHOSPHORUS-32 (^{32}P)

Phosphorus-32 localises in bone marrow or trabecular or cortical bone depending on the chemical form of ^{32}P used. A low tumour to normal bone ratio of only 2:1 is unacceptable from a therapeutic standpoint as it leads to severe toxicity from marrow suppression (30-40%). A number of different methods have been used to enhance tumour uptake, including androgen priming[10] and parathyroid hormone administration[11]. Using these manipulations pain relief has been reported in 50-87% of patients using daily injections of 40-80 MBq ^{32}P to a dose of 200-400 MBq[10]. Severe toxic side-effects have been reported, however, with a high incidence of myelosuppression.

References

1. Stoll BA. Natural history, prognosis and staging of bone metastases pp1-4 in Stoll BA and Parbhoo S (eds) Bone Metastases monitoring and treatment, New York, *Raven* 1983.

2. Robinson RG, Spicer JA, Preston DF, Wegst AV, Martin NL. Treatment of metastatic bone pain with 89-Strontium. *Int J Rad Appl Instrum* (B) 1987; **1**: 219-222.

3. Laing AH, Ackery DM, Bayly RJ, Buchanan RB, Lewington VJ, McEwan AJ, Mcleod PM, Zivanovic MA. Strontium-89 therapy for pain palliation in prostatic skeletal malignancy. *Br J Radiol* 1991; **64**: 816-822.

4. Lewington VJ, McEwan AJ, Ackery DM, Bayly RJ, Keeling DH, Macleod PM, Porter AT, Zivanovic MA. A prospective randomised double blind crossover study to examine the efficacy of strontium-89 in pain palliation in patients with advanced prostate cancer metastatic to bone. *Eur J Cancer* 1991; **27**: 954-958.

5. Ksai LP, Fossella F, Holoye P, Podoloff D, Kim E, Crane J, Gordon EE. Evaluation of multiple dose Sm-153 EDTMP for bone pain palliation in cancer patients. Proc 7th International symposium of radiopharmacy *Bostn, Mass.* 1991; p11.

6. Turner JH, Claringbod PG. A phase II study of the treatment of painful multifocal bone metastases with single and repeated doses of Sm-153-EDTMP. *Eur. J. Cancer* 1991; **27**: 1084-1086.

7. Maxon HR, Schroder LE, Thomas SR. Re-186(Sn)HEDP for treatment of painful osseous metastases: initial clinical experience on 20 patients with hormone resistant prostate cancer. *Radiology* 1990; **176**: 155-159.

8. Maxon HR, Schroder LE, Hertzberg VS, Thomas SR, Englaro EE, Samaratunga R, Smith H, Moulton JS, Williams CC, Erhardt GH, Schneider HJ. Rhenium 186-(Sn) HEDP for treatment of painful osseous metastases: results of a double blind crossover trial, comparison with placebo. *J. Nuclear Medicine.* 1991; **32**: 1877-1881.

9. Zonnenberg BA, de Klerk JMH, van Rijk PP, Quirijnen JM, van het Schip AD, van Dijk A, ten Kroode NF. Re-186 HEDP for treatment of painful bone metastases in patients with metastatic prostate or breast cancer. Preliminary results. *J. of Nuclear Medicine* 1991; **32**: 1082.

10. Burnet NG, Williams G, Howard N. Phosphorus 32 for intractable bone pain from carcinoma of the prostate. *Clin. Oncol.* 1990; **2**: 220-223.

11. Tong ECK. Parathormone and P-32 therapy in prostate cancer with bone metastases. *Radiology* 1971; **98**: 343-351.

Regionally Localised Radionuclide Therapy

INTRODUCTION

One of the major problems with radionuclide therapy is the toxicity to normal tissues. When the radiopharmaceutical is introduced directly into the locality of the tumour, high concentrations of the radiopharmaceutical will result. This regional localisation of the radiopharmaceutical may be achieved by direct intravascular (intra-arterial or intralymphatic), intracavitary (pericardial, pleural or peritoneal) or intralesional administration.

INTRAVASCULAR ADMINISTRATION
Intra-arterial

Direct injection of a therapeutic radiopharmaceutical into the vascular bed perfusing a tumour will result in high concentrations of the agent provided it undergoes extensive deposition in the vascular bed of the tumour. The results of intra-arterial injection are improved by selecting a radiopharmaceutical that either temporarily or permanently occludes the vascular bed. This form of therapy is most effective against small volume tumours with small vascular beds.

An area where arterial infusion therapy has proved most effective is in the liver where this technique can be used to treat unresectable tumours. To avoid systemic distribution of the agent, the shunt volume should be low. This can be assessed prior to therapy using ^{99m}Tc albumen microspheres.

The agents commonly used are ^{131}I-Lipiodol and ^{131}I-Ethiodol. Doses of 74 MBq to 4.4 GBq have been used, resulting in tumour shrinkage and palliation. As some lung deposition of radiopharmaceutical is observed, ceramic, resin and glass microspheres have been developed labelled with ^{32}P or ^{90}Y. Careful incorporation of the radiolabel into the microsphere is now performed to avoid the unwanted dissociation of the therapeutic radionuclide from the microsphere with subsequent systemic distribution. Care in positioning the catheter tip prior to injection is also vital to avoid normal tissue damage.

Side-effects of fever, elevation of liver enzymes and abdominal discomfort have been reported[1].

Response rates of up to 75% have been reported in hepatocellular cancer and hepatic metastases[2], but no definite prolongation of survival has been demonstrated.

Intralymphatic

Although several reports of the use of ^{131}I-Lipiodol (20 MBq) mixed with ^{32}P-tri-n-octyl-phosphate (80 MBq) in the treatment of micrometastases in patients with malignant melanoma have appeared in the literature, the contraindications of lymphatic blockage and large-volume disease significantly limit clinical studies.

INTRACAVITARY ADMINISTRATION
Intrapericardial

The successful use of ^{32}P-colloid (185-1100 MBq) in patients with malignant pericardial effusions has been reported[3] in 40% of patients. The treatment is well tolerated, with problems of pericarditis only reported after repeat treatments.

Intrapleural

Palliative therapy using 220-370 MBq of ^{32}P or 2.5-4.0 GBq ^{90}Y mixed with saline in patients with malignant effusions has been found to stop effusion formation in 50 -75% of patients. A tracer dose of radiopharmaceutical should be administered prior to treatment to ensure distribution of radiopharmaceutical throughout the pleural cavity[4]. No improvement in survival rate has thus far been documented. No side-effects from treatment have been recorded.

Intraperitoneal

The therapeutic installation of ^{32}P-colloid or ^{90}Y in saline into the peritoneal cavity is the most commonly performed technique of intracavitary therapy. Its main use is in the treatment of ovarian cancer, when it can be used as adjuvant therapy following surgery for the primary tumour or recurrence. It may also be used as an adjuvant to chemotherapy. The addition of radionuclide therapy to chemotherapy improves the 4-year survival rate from 22% with chemotherapy alone to 59% with combination therapy[5].

Doses of ^{32}P used range from 370 MBq to 4.0 GBq and the dose ranges for ^{90}Y-colloid are 2.5-4.0 GBq. The response rate appears to be dose dependent. This therapy may also be used to treat patients with malignant ascites, the success rate being 85%.

Side-effects are few, although patients treated with gold-198 have experienced severe ileus.

INTRACYSTIC ADMINISTRATION

Radionuclide therapy has been used to treat cystic intracerebral tumours in order to prevent fluid accumulation within the cystic lesion. The beta radiation delivered directly into the cyst enables high doses of radiation to be administered with sparing of adjacent normal tissue.

The radiopharmaceuticals used are colloids labelled with ^{32}P, ^{90}Y and ^{186}Re. Doses administered depend on the volume of the cyst and range from 18-56 MBq in craniopharyngiomas and from 4-90 MBq in cystic astrocytomas[6]. Results reported are superior to those for the intracystic administration of chemotherapeutic agents or sclerosants. The results are long-lived and accompanied by few side-effects, although fits have been rarely reported.

Solid lesions and lesions with mixed cystic and solid components are not amenable to this therapy[7].

References

1. Gross-Fengels W, Fischbach R, Lackner K, Zieren U, Chemoembolisation (CHe) von Lebermalignomen: Ansprechraten und Uberlebenszeiten. *Zbl Rad* 1992; **146:** 64.

2. Shapiro B, Andres J, Figg L, Carey J, Walker-Andrews S, Smith J, Ensminger W. Therapeutic intraarterial administration of yttrium-90 glass microspheres for hepatic tumours. *European J. of Nuclear Medicine* 1989; **8:** 401

3. Firusian N. ^{32}P therapy for malignant pericardial effusion. *Onkologie* 1991; **3:** 12-17.

4. Askienazy S, Turak B, Piketty ML, Munari C, Habert MD, Lebtahi R, Dilouya A, Chodkiewicz JP. Colloidal ^{186}Re in the intracavitary irradiation of cystic craniopharyngiomas. *J. of Nuclear Medicine* 1990; **31:** S143.

5. Hoefnagel CA. Radionuclide therapy revisited. *European J. of Nuclear Medicine* 1991; **18:** 408-431.

6. Shapiro B, Fig LM, Carey J, Kallus M, Taren J, Hood T. Intracavitary therapy of cystic brain tumours with ^{32}P chromic phosphate colloid. In: Schmidt HAE and Chambron J (eds) Nuclear medicine quantitative analysis in imaging and function *Stuttgart Schattauer* 1990; 574-576.

7. Bernstein M, Gutin PH. Interstitial irradiation of skull base tumours. *Can. J. Neurol. Sci.* 1985; **12:** 366-370.

Radionuclide Therapy Using Monoclonal Antibodies

Monoclonal antibodies targeting tumour-specific antigens on cell surfaces offer potential new therapeutic agents in a wide variety of tumours. The results of phase II and phase III trials have so far been disappointing in solid tumours. Exceptions are radiosensitive tumours such as lymphoma[1,2,3] and where intra-cavitary[4,5,6], intra-arterial[7] or intra-tumoral[8] administration of the radiolabelled antibody has been performed.

The reasons for the poor results in solid tumours treated intravenously are mainly the low uptake of the radiolabelled antibody, which may be less than 0.01% of the injected dose per gram of tumour, and the non-homogeneous distribution of the antibody within the tumour. However, the uptake of chemotherapeutic agents may be even less as they are not usually selectively taken up by the cancer. At present minimal residual disease is the best target for radio-immuno therapy in solid tumours [9].

Several new approaches are currently being evaluated. The dose delivered to the tumour target may theoretically be increased by improving the tumour blood flow, by increasing the expression of antigenic sites at the surface of the tumour or by prolonging the residence time of the radionuclide in the tumour.

Two-stage pretargeting has also been explored as a method of reducing the delivery of radiolabelled antibody to normal tissues. This has been achieved using bispecific antibody, antibody conjugated with avidin or biotin, antibody conjugated with an oligonucleotide and a radiolabelled antisense oligonucleotide and finally using antibody conjugated with an enzyme and a radiolabelled enzymic inhibitor.

References

1. De Nardo SJ, de Nardo GL, O'Grady LF. Treatment of a patient with a B cell lymphoma by ^{131}I LYM-1 monoclonal antibodies. *Int. J. of Biological Markers* 1987; **2**: 49-53.

2. Kaminsky MS, Zasadny KR, Francis IR et al. Radioimmunotherapy of B-cell lymphoma with ^{131}I] anti-B1 (anti-CD20) antibody. *New England J. of Medicine* 1993; **329**: 459-465.

3. Press OW, Eary JF, Appelbaum FR et al. Radiolabelled-antibody therapy of B-cell lymphoma with autologous bone marrow support. *New England J. of Medicine* 1993; **329**: 1219-1224.

4. Ward BJ, Mather SJ, Hawkins L. Localisation of radioiodine conjugated to the monoclonal antibody HMFG2 in human ovarian cancer: assessment of intravenous and intraperitoneal routes of administration. *Cancer Research* 1987; **47**: 4719-4723

5. Stuart JS, Hird V, Snook D et al. Intraperitoneal radioimmunotherapy for ovarian cancer: pharmacokinetics, toxicity and efficacy of I-131 labelled monoclonal antibodies. *Int. J. Radiation Oncol. Biol. Phys.* 1989; **16**: 405-413.

6. Stuart JS, Hird V, Snook D et al. Intraperitoneal yttrium-90-labelled monoclonal antibody in ovarian cancer. *J. of Clin. Oncol.* 1990; **8**: 1941-1950.

7. Delaloye B, Bischof-Delaloye A, Volant J. First approach to therapy of liver metastases in colorectal cancer by intrahepatically infused ^{131}I labelled monoclonal anti CEA antibodies. *European J. of Nuclear Medicine* 1985; **11**: A11.

8. Riva P, Arista A, Sturiale C et al. Treatment of intracranial human glioblastoma by direct intratumoral administration of ^{131}I-labelled anti-tenascin monoclonal antibody BC-2. *Int. J. of Cancer* 1992; **51**: 7-13.

9. Bischof-Delaloye A, Delaloye B. Radiolabelled monoclonal antibodies in tumour imaging and therapy: out of fashion? *European J. of Nuclear Medicine* 1995; **22**: 571-580.

Evaluation of Effects of Cancer Therapy on Organ Function

INTRODUCTION

Chemotherapy and radiotherapy can produce a variety of acute and chronic organ toxicities. These organ toxicities may be acute and may produce life-threatening problems, such as hypotension, respiratory distress and renal failure.

These reactions may necessitate tapering or cessation of treatment with the particular drug. If the offending drug is discontinued at an early stage, the manifestations of toxicity usually subside. The initial manifestations of organ injury are usually functional. Thus, nuclear medicine techniques, which predominantly provide functional information, are particularly well suited to detect these adverse events at an early stage[1].

CARDIOTOXICITY

In cancer patients undergoing therapy, the cardiac status occasionally requires evaluation[2,3]; this is especially so in patients who have received doxorubicin, which is an important cause of cardiomyopathy. This medication is extremely useful in the treatment of many neoplastic diseases. However, a cumulative dose-related myopathy develops in some 2% of patients, usually when cumulative doses reach 400 mg/kg and the figure increases to 20% with cumulative doses of 700 mg/kg[4], thus limiting further use of the drug and effective treatment of the tumour. Patients receiving doses in this range should have their cardiac ejection fraction (EF) evaluated prior to further therapy. Cardiotoxicity should be suspected if the EF falls below 45% or by 5% on sequential scans. Anthracycline derivatives such as epirubicin and mitoxantrone have a lesser degree of cardiotoxicity. Other antineoplastic drugs also exert cardiotoxic effects and

Doxorubicin	Ifosfamide
Mitoxantrone	Epirubicin
Cyclophosphamide	Taxol
Vincristine	5-Fluorouracil
Cisplatin	Interferon
Amsacrine	

Table 16.1 *Antitumour drugs that may produce cardiotoxicity*

these are listed in Table 16.1.

Radiation-induced cardiac damage may lead to pericarditis and myocarditis. The incidence of pericarditis depends upon volume and dose of radiation and is generally 2.5% if the pericardium is excluded from the field. Pericarditis occurs at an early stage (within a few weeks), while myocarditis is a slow process and has a latency of several years. In patients undergoing mediastinal irradiation the ejection fraction falls in the first 2 weeks and recovers by 2 months.

Other radiopharmaceuticals which can be used to assess cardiac injury are ^{111}In-antimyocin (Fab) and ^{123}I-MIBG[1]. ^{111}In–antimyocin (Fab) is a radiolabelled MoAb fragment which binds to intracellular myocin filaments when sarcolemmal disruption occurs. This helps to identify sites of injury secondary to drug toxicity. The uptake of this tracer is diffuse and appears to precede left ventricular ejection fraction deterioration. It is also possible to evaluate myocardial adrenergic damage by using ^{123}I-MIBG. Damage to the neurones results in diffuse and decreased uptake of ^{123}I-MIBG.

Kidney

The kidneys are responsible for elimination of many chemotherapeutic drugs and their metabolites and therefore are more vulnerable to injury. For example, cisplatin and ifosfamide are two cytoxic drugs which can lead to progressive dose-related deterioration of renal function[5]. Other antineoplastic drugs which cause nephrotoxicity are listed in Table 16.2. The toxicity is generally dose-related and can involve any part of the nephron. Glomerular filtration rate (GFR) measurements are frequently used to monitor

114

Cisplatin	Ifosfamide
Methotrexate (in high doses)	Mitomycin
Diaziquone (in high doses)	Azacitidine
Pentostatin	Plicamycin
Streptozocin	Interleukin-2

Table 16.2 *Chemotherapeutic agents that have a high potential for nephrotoxicity*

nephrotoxicity. Accurate measurements of the GFR can be obtained using chromium-51 ethylene diamine tetra-acetic acid (^{51}Cr-EDTA) clearance. This test is simple, fairly rigorous and useful for serial monitoring of renal function. Other measures of renal function such as plasma creatinine are dependent on non-renal factors such as rate of creatinine generation (dependent on muscle mass) and extrarenal elimination. This measure is particularly inappropriate in children with cancer, especially when they are cachectic. Measures of creatinine clearance can also be used to monitor renal function, but caution needs to be exercised mainly because of the effects of tubular secretion, especially when the GFR falls. The error induced by this measure may be a twofold or greater overestimate of the true value.

Renal blood flow and function can also be monitored by sequential renography at regular intervals to detect onset of obstruction to outflow or to evaluate renal toxicity. For imaging ^{99m}Tc-diethylene triamine penta-acetic acid (^{99m}Tc–DTPA), ^{99m}Tc-mercaptoacetyltriglycine (^{99m}Tc-MAG3) and ^{99m}Tc-DMSA may be used. Obstructive nephropathy in cancer patients is usually secondary to fibrosis, particularly in patients with ovarian and cervical cancers who have undergone radical pelvic surgery, radiotherapy and/or chemotherapy. Unilateral renal damage secondary to irradiation can also be measured with ^{99m}Tc-DMSA, which gives fairly accurate divided function[1].

BOWEL DAMAGE

Bowel irradiation can cause acute and delayed toxic events. Acute toxicity results in nausea and vomiting and nuclear medicine has no role in these. Delayed toxic events usually occur between 6 and 24 months with an incidence of 1–10%. Diarrhoea is the most common presenting symptom and is frequently caused by bile acid malabsorption as a result of terminal ileitis or ileal resection. However, diarrhoea may be caused by intraluminal bacterial overgrowth due to stasis. Bile acid malabsorbtion may be tested using ^{75}Se-HCAT. This is a taurine conjugate of a synthetic bile acid (23 selena 25 homotaurocholate) labelled with ^{75}Se. In patients with bile acid malabsorption ^{75}Se–HCAT retention is significantly reduced. The combination of ^{75}Se-HCAT test with one of bacterial colonization (e.g. ^{14}C breath test or Schilling's test) helps to establish whether diarrhoea is related to bile acid malabsorption, bacterial overgrowth or other non–ileal causes[1].

LUNG DAMAGE

Radiation pneumonitis and lung fibrosis are occasional sequelae of cancer therapy. Radiation pneumonitis may occur 2-6 months post irradiation and may subsequently lead to fibrosis. ^{67}Ga scintigraphy is useful to monitor these changes. Generally increased tracer uptake is noted in the irradiated field during the early phase. If no treatment is given for pneumonitis the scans return to normal by 5-6 months; however, if steroids are given then the response is more rapid. Diffuse bilateral lung uptake outside the field of irradiation is a poor prognostic indicator[6].

Chemotherapy-related lung toxicity is uncommon. Bleomycin is most commonly associated with lung toxicity; especially when given in combination with nitrosurea it may lead to pulmonary fibrosis in the late period. Lung toxicity with both drugs is dose dependent. Other chemotherapeutic agents which may cause lung toxicity include cyclophosphamide, busulphan and methotrexate.

MISCELLANEOUS TOXICITIES

Other organs such as brain, salivary glands, liver, bone and bone marrow can all be affected by the toxic effects of antineoplastic therapy. The value of routine use of nuclear medicine investigations to monitor these adverse effects is less clear and is discussed extensively by Valdes Olmos et al.[1].

References

1. Olmos RAV, Hoefnagel CA, van der Schoot JB. Nuclear medicine in the monitoring of organ function and the detection of injury. *European J. of Nuclear Medicine* 1993; **20**: 515-546.

2. Pryor DB, Harrell FE.Jr, Lee KL et al. Prognostic indicators from radionuclide angiography in medically treated patients with coronary artery disease. *Am. J. of Cardiology* 1984; **53**: 18-22.

3. Iskandrian AS, Hakki AH, Goel IP et al. The use of rest and exercise radionuclide ventriculography in risk stratification in patients with suspected coronary artery disease. *Am. Heart J.* 1985; **110**: 864-872.

4. Alexander J, Dainiak N, Berger HJ et al. Serial assessment of doxorubicin cardiotoxicity with quantitative radionuclide angiography. *New England J. of Medicine* 1979; **300**: 278-283.

5. Pratt CB, Meyer WH, Jenkins JJ et al. Ifosfamide, Fanconi's syndrome, and rickets. *J. of Clin. Oncology* 1991; **9**: 1495-1499.

6. Katoka M, Kawamura M, Itoh H, Hamamoto K. Ga-67 citrate scintigraphy for the early detection of radiation pneumonitis. *Clinical Nuclear Medicine* 1992; **17**: 27-31.